A Psychiatric Glossary

*The meaning of words
most frequently used
in psychiatry*

Second Edition

by the

COMMITTEE ON PUBLIC INFORMATION
AMERICAN PSYCHIATRIC ASSOCIATION

Washington, D. C. — 1964

first edition   May 1957

second edition   April 1964

published by   AMERICAN PSYCHIATRIC ASSOCIATION
1700 18th St., N.W.
Washington, D. C. 20009

PRESENTING THE SECOND EDITION

The American Psychiatric Association takes pride in presenting this new edition of *A Psychiatric Glossary* in the wake of a first edition which proved so useful to scores of thousands of people.

A comparison of the new with the old edition reflects the general lines of advance in psychiatry over the past decade. In 1957, when the first edition appeared, the new psychotropic drugs had just established themselves in the psychiatric armamentarium and their tremendous potential was not clearly perceived. While research in the neurophysiology and biochemistry of mental illness was considered promising, their terminology was not sufficiently in circulation to justify inclusion in a popular glossary. The old-fashioned terms associated with mental deficiency remained in vogue. While one spoke loosely at the time of "community psychiatry," the definitive work of the *Joint Commission on Mental Illness and Health* was barely under way, and no one at the time would have dreamed that its bold recommendations for a national community mental health program would have the unequivocal support of a President of the United States, John Fitzgerald Kennedy, and the U.S. Congress.

All of these developments are accounted for in the many new words in this volume. The Committee's effort to bring its definitions into closer accord with the official *Diagnostic and Statistical Manual for Mental Disorders* further serves the interest of clarity. Many other minor improvements in style are to be noted.

May we look forward to a third edition some years hence which will reflect as much progress! The Committee on Public Information deserves the Association's thanks for a job well done. Those who thought so highly of the first edition should doubly welcome the second.

Jack R. Ewalt, M.D., *President*

Boston, Massachusetts
March, 1964

INTRODUCTION

This Glossary traces its inception to the Annual Meeting of the American Psychiatric Association in 1952. At that time several science writers in attendance urged that a popular glossary would not only help reporters but would also contribute to clarifying widespread misconceptions of psychiatric words and concepts. With this encouragement, the Committee on Public Information asked, and received, permission from the Association's governing Council to proceed. The work began that year.

In retrospect it is fair to venture that the Committee would have been delighted had the first edition sold as many as 5,000 copies. It has been a matter of continuous astonishment that in a seven-year span about 160,000 copies have been sold and that it has continued to sell at the rate of about 1,000 copies a month until the 12th printing was exhausted this past month.

The readership has been largely concentrated in the medical profession and the mental health disciplines of psychology, social work, and nursing, especially student nurses. At one point, by courtesy of a pharmaceutical manufacturer, 50,000 copies were distributed to general physicians throughout the country to further the broad effort to bring them into closer rapport with psychiatry. It has been especially gratifying that secretarial personnel in all kinds of psychiatric facilities have found it helpful. It is a curious and somewhat amusing tribute that the familiar cover of the book is frequently seen jutting from the coat pockets of aspiring candidates at the time of their examinations by the American Board of Psychiatry and Neurology. Undergraduate medical students, various kinds of activity therapists in psychiatric treatment centers, psychiatric aides, lawyers, school teachers, public health workers, clergymen, and others in substantial numbers have found it useful.

The second edition, like the first, has been approximately five years in the making. Mindful of Shakespeare's caution that "words without thoughts never to Heaven go," the Committee leans to the view that the better part of a decade should pass between new editions. Each year, professional literature produces a new crop of words, many of them coined by authors for an *ad hoc* purpose. Some stand the test of time. Most do not. A suitable "wait and see" period seems in order.

The first edition of the *Glossary* contained somewhat fewer than 500 entries. The new one contains nearly 700, of which approximately 150 are new terms derived primarily from psychopharmacology, neurophysiology, biochemistry, mental retardation, and community psychiatry. Several other words from "dynamic psychiatry," omitted in the first edition, are present in the second; and about a dozen others have been deleted because their meaning was so self-evident. It is of some interest that fewer than 100 definitions in the first edition survived in their original form in the final copy for the second edition.

By way of expressing appreciation to those who contributed to the *Glossary,* the first edition noted that many hundreds of Fellows and Members of the Association had reviewed and criticized various drafts. Thanks to them must be repeated, for the new is built on the foundations of the old. This new volume, however, is largely the work of the present members of the Committee whose names appear on the page opposite, and most especially of our beloved Chairman, the late Robert T. Morse, M.D., to whom this work is affectionately dedicated. Finally, a special word of appreciation to Robert L. Robinson, the Association's Public Information Officer since 1948. What was said of him in the introduction in the first edition is even more pertinent today: "He kept us in motion, pricked our consciences when we sought refuge in professional jargon, and helped resolve many thorny problems of terminology."

Zigmond M. Lebensohn, M.D., *Chairman*
Commitee on Public Information

April 1964

ACKNOWLEDGMENTS

PRESIDENTS OF THE ASSOCIATION 1952-1964

D. Ewen Cameron, M.D., 1952-1953
Kenneth E. Appel, M.D., 1953-1954
Arthur P. Noyes, M.D., 1954-1955
R. Finley Gayle, Jr., M.D., 1955-1956
Francis J. Braceland, M.D., 1956-1957
Harry C. Solomon, M.D., 1957-1958
Francis J. Gerty, M.D., 1958-1959
William Malamud, M.D., 1959-1960
Robert H. Felix, M.D., 1960-1961
Walter E. Barton, M.D., 1961-1962
C. H. Hardin Branch, M.D., 1962-1963
Jack R. Ewalt, M.D., 1963-1964
Daniel Blain, M.D., 1964-1965

THE COMMITTEE ON PUBLIC INFORMATION 1952-1964

*Wilfred Bloomberg, M.D., *Chairman,* 1951-1955
Edward G. Billings, M.D.
Rives Chalmers, M.D.
Nicholas P. Dallis, M.D.
Edward M. Daniels, M.D.
J. Lawrence Evans, M.D.
David J. Flicker, M.D.
Irving A. Gail, M.D.
Edward O. Harper, M.D.
*L. Lee Hasenbush, M.D.
Robert O. Jones, M.D.
Henry P. Laughlin, M.D., *Chairman,* 1957-1961
*Zigmond M. Lebensohn, M.D., *Chairman,* 1964-
*Burness Moore, M.D.
*Robert T. Morse, M.D., *Chairman,* 1955-1957, 1961-
   1964. Deceased, February 18, 1964.
J. Martin Myers, M.D.
*Myrick W. Pullen, Jr., M.D.
*C. A. Roberts, M.D.
Marvin Stern, M.D.
*David A. Young, M.D.
            *Indicates present members

CHAIRMEN OF THE COORDINATING COMMITTEE ON COMMUNITY ASPECTS OF PSYCHIATRY

William C. Menninger, M.D., 1952-1957
Paul V. Lemkau, M.D., 1957-1963
Milton Greenblatt, 1963-

PUBLIC INFORMATION OFFICE

Walter E. Barton, M.D., Medical Director
Robert L. Robinson, M.A., Public Information Officer

Dedicated to

ROBERT THATCHER MORSE, M.D.

1905 - 1964

In Affectionate Memory

TO THE READER:

Nearly all words which are printed in *italics* are defined in this glossary for convenient cross reference. Sometimes the abbreviation *q.v.* is used to encourage the reader to cross-check one reference with another.

a

abreaction: Emotional release or discharge resulting from recalling to awareness a painful experience which has been forgotten (repressed) because it was consciously intolerable. Its therapeutic effect occurs through discharge of the painful emotions, desensitization to them, and often, increased insight.

accident prone: In psychiatry, special susceptibility to accidents due to psychological causes.

acrophobia: See *phobia.*

acting out: Expression of unconscious emotional conflicts or feelings of hostility or love in actions that the protagonist does not consciously know are related to such conflicts or feelings. May be harmful or, in controlled situations, therapeutic (e.g. children's play therapy).

acute situational or stress reaction: See *gross stress reaction.*

addiction: Strong emotional and/or psychological dependence upon a substance, such as alcohol or a drug, which has progressed beyond voluntary control.

adjustment: The relation between the individual, his inner self, and his environment.

Adler, Alfred (1870-1937): Viennese psychiatrist. See *individual psychology, inferiority complex* (under *complex*), *compensation* and *overcompensation.*

adrenergic: Activated or transmitted by adrenalin (e.g. *sympathetic nerve fibers*). See also *sympathetic nervous system.*

aerophagia: Excessive or morbid air swallowing.

9

affect: A person's emotional feeling tone. Affect and emotion are commonly used interchangeably.

affective psychosis: A psychotic reaction in which the predominant feature is a severe disorder of mood or emotional feelings. In general, equivalent to *manic depressive reaction* (q.v.).

aggression: In psychiatry, forceful attacking action, physical, verbal or symbolic. May be realistic and self-protective, including healthful self-assertiveness; may be unrealistic and directed outwardly toward environment or inwardly toward self.

>**constructive aggression:** Self-protective and preservative; realistically evoked by threats from others; includes healthful self-assertiveness which is necessary to protect one's reasonable rights.

>**destructive aggression:** Not realistically essential for self-preservation or protection.

>**inward aggression:** Directed toward the self.

agitated depression: A psychotic depression accompanied by continuous restlessness. See *depression*.

agitation: State of chronic restlessness; a major psycho-motor expression of emotional tension.

agnosia: Inability to recognize and interpret the significance of sensory impressions due to organic brain disorder.

agoraphobia: See *phobia*.

ailurophobia: See *phobia*.

akathisia: Originally, a difficulty in sitting down. More recently broadened to include restlessness and uncontrolled muscular movements, sometimes seen as side effects in the use of certain psychotropic drugs, such as the *phenothiazines* (q.v.).

alcoholic psychoses: a group of severe mental disorders, associated with brain damage or dysfunction, resulting from excessive use of alcohol. See also *psychosis*.

Alcoholics Anonymous (A.A.): The name of a group composed of former alcoholics who collectively assist alcoholics through personal and group support.

alcoholism: The overuse of alcohol to the extent of habituation, dependence, or addiction. Alcoholism is medically sigificant when it impairs or threatens physical or mental health, or when it hampers personal relationships and individual effectiveness.

algophobia: See *phobia*.

alienist: Obsolete legal term for a psychiatrist who testifies in court as to a person's sanity and mental competence.

Alzheimer's disease: A degenerative organic brain disease generally occurring in middle life. Similar to *Pick's disease* (q.v.).

ambivalence: The coexistence of two opposing drives, desires, feelings or emotions toward the same person, object or goal. These may be conscious or partly conscious; or one side of the feelings may be unconscious. Example: love and hate toward the same person.

ambulatory schizophrenia: See under *schizophrenia*.

amentia: An old term meaning absence of intellect as in severe congenital *mental retardation* (q.v.). The basis of amentia is usually organic and due to a developmental lack of adequate brain tissue. To be distinguished from *dementia* (q.v.).

American Board of Psychiatry and Neurology: An incorporated certifying body of representatives appointed by the American Medical Association, American Neurological Association, and American Psychiatric Association. Founded in 1934. It conducts examinations and certifies successful candidates as "Diplomates"—i.e. qualified specialists in psychiatry and/or neurology.

American Psychiatric Association: Leading national professional organization in the United States for physicians who specialize in psychiatry. Also includes members from Canada, Central America and the Caribbean Islands, and Corresponding Members from other countries. Founded in 1844 as the Association of Medical Superintendents of American Institutions for the Insane. The name was changed to American Medico-Psychological Association in 1891 and to its present designation in 1921. In 1964 the membership was approximately 14,000.

amines: Organic compounds containing the amino group $(-NH_2)$. Of special importance in biochemistry and neurochemistry. See also *biogenic amines* and *catecholamines*.

11

amnesia: Pathological loss of memory; forgetting; a phenom enon in which an area of one's experience or recollections is forgotten and becomes consciously inaccessible. It may be of organic, emotional, or mixed origin, and sharply circum scribed in limits of time.

amphetamines: A group of antidepressant chemicals which produce a temporary feeling of well-being by cortical stimu lation.

anaclitic: Leaning on. In psychoanalytic terminology, de notes dependence of the infant on the mother or mother sub stitute for his sense of well being (e.g. gratification through nursing). Normal in childhood; pathologic in later years if excessive.

anaclitic depression: An acute and striking impairment of an infant's physical, social, and intellectual development which sometimes occurs following a sudden separation from the mothering person. See also *depression*.

anal character: In psychoanalysis, a pattern of behavior in an adult which originates in the *anal erotism* of infancy (q.v.) and which is characterized by such traits as excessive order liness, miserliness, obstinacy, etc. "Anal" traits in moder ate degree are normal; in excessive degree they predispose to the development of *obsessive-compulsive* symptoms (q.v.).

anal erotism: Pleasurable part of the experience of anal function. In later life anal erotism usually appears in dis guised and sublimated forms. See also: *erotic; sublimation.*

analgesia: A state in which the sense of pain is lulled or stopped.

analysand: A patient in psychoanalytic treatment.

analysis: A common synonym for *psychoanalysis* (q.v.).

analytic psychology: The name given by the Swiss psycho analyst, Carl Gustav Jung (1875-1961) to his theoretical sys tem which minimizes the influence of sexual factors in emo tional disorders and stresses mystical religious factors. See also *Jung.*

analyzer: A term used in Pavlovian theory to include the external sense organs and their cerebral connections.

anamnesis: The developmental history of an individual and of his illness, especially a patient's recollections.

anesthesia: The state of having no feeling. In surgical procedures the process of inducing unconsciousness by use of medication. In neurology, the lack of sensation after nerve damage. In *conversion reaction* (q.v. under *psychoneurosis*) or *hypnosis,* the same apparent lack of sensation, without damage, due to a psychic process.

anhedonia: Chronic inability to experience pleasure. See also *hedonism.*

anima: In Jungian psychology, the inner being of an individual as opposed to the outer character or *persona* (q.v.) which he presents to the world. Further, the *anima* may be the more feminine *soul* or inner self of a man; the *animus* the more masculine *soul* of a woman. See also *Jung.*

anorexia nervosa: A syndrome marked by severe and prolonged loss of appetite with marked weight loss and other symptoms resulting from emotional conflict. Most frequently encountered in young females.

anti-depressant: Popular term for various groups of drugs used in treating depressions. Not to be confused with *tranquilizers* or *ataractics* (q.v.).

anxiety: Apprehension, tension or uneasiness which stems from the anticipation of danger, the source of which is largely unknown or unrecognized. Primarily of intrapsychic origin, in distinction to fear, which is the emotional response to a consciously recognized and usually external threat or danger. Anxiety and fear are accompanied by similar physiologic changes. May be regarded as pathologic when present to such extent as to interfere with effectiveness in living, achievement of desired goals or satisfactions, or reasonable emotional comfort.

anxiety hysteria: Primarily a psychoanalytic term for a neurosis characterized by *anxiety* (q.v.) and *phobic reactions* (q.v.). Not to be confused with *hysteria* (q.v.).

anxiety neurosis: Anxiety reaction. See under *psychoneurosis.*

aphasia: Disturbance of speech due to organic brain disease and manifested by loss of ability to pronounce words, or to name common objects and indicate their use correctly. In **motor aphasia** understanding remains but the ability to speak is lost. In **sensory aphasia** the ability to comprehend the meaning of words or phrases or the use of objects is lost.

aphonia: Inability to produce normal speech sounds. May be due either to organic or psychic causes.

apperception: Perception as modified and enhanced by the individual's own emotions, memories and biases.

association: Relationship between ideas or emotions by contiguity, continuity, or by similarities. See also *free association*.

asthenia: Weakness.

asylum: Obsolete term for mental hospital.

ataractic: A recent term for drugs used to decrease anxiety. Essentially, the same as *tranquilizers*.

atypical child: Nonspecific term for a child with distorted personality development. Applied most often to *autistic children* (q.v.) with perceptual handicaps and brain damage.

aura: In epilepsy, a premonitory, subjective sensation (e.g. a flash of light) which often warns the patient of an impending convulsion.

autism (autistic thinking): A form of thinking which gratifies unfulfilled desires without regard for reality. Objective facts are distorted, obscured, or excluded in varying degree.

early infantile autism (Kanner's syndrome): A term used in child psychiatry to refer to babies who remain aloof from relationships with others, but usually without evidence of intellectual impairment.

autistic child: In child psychiatry, a child who responds chiefly to inner thoughts, who does not relate to his environment, and whose over-all functioning is immature and often appears retarded. May be an extension of *early infantile autism* (q.v). Often used interchangeably with *childhood schizophrenia* (q.v.).

autoerotism: Sensual self-gratification from one's self. Characteristic of, but not limited to, an early stage of emotional development. Includes satisfactions deriving from genital play, masturbation, and from oral, anal, visual sources and fantasy.

automatism: Automatic and apparently undirected symbolic behavior which is not consciously controlled. See also *schizophrenia, dissociative reactions* and *epilepsy*.

utonomic nervous system: That part of the nervous system rdinarily not subject to voluntary control. It operates outide of consciousness and controls basic life preserving funcions such as the heart rate and breathing.

b

Beers, Clifford W. (1876-1943): Author of *A Mind That Found Itself* and founder in 1909 of the *National Committee for Mental Hygiene,* now the *National Association for Mental Health.*

behaviorism: A body of psychologic theory developed by *John B. Watson* (1878-1958), concerned chiefly with objectively observable, tangible, and measurable data, rather than with subjective phenomena such as ideas and emotions.

belle indifférence: Literally, "beautiful indifference." Seen in certain patients with somatic conversion (hysteria); describes patients with inappropriate lack of concern for the implications of their disability. See also *conversion reaction* under *psychoneurosis.*

bestiality: Sexual relations between human and animal.

biogenic amines: A group of amines formed in the living organism, some of which exert an important influence on nervous system activity. Examples: *epinephrine, norepinephrine* and *serotonin*.

birth trauma: Term used by *Otto Rank* (1844-1939) to relate his theories of anxiety and neurosis to the inevitable psychic shock of being born.

Bleuler, Eugen (1857-1939): Eminent Swiss psychiatrist whose investigation of *dementia praecox* led him to the alternate term *schizophrenia*, now in common usage. His studies enriched the concept of this disorder.

blocking: Difficulty in recollection, or interruption of a train of thought or speech, due to emotional factors usually unconscious.

body image: The conscious and unconscious picture a person has of his body at any moment. The conscious and unconscious images may differ from each other.

borderline state (borderline psychosis): A diagnostic term used when it is difficult to determine whether symptoms are predominantly neurotic or psychotic. The symptoms may shift quickly from one pattern to another. They are frequently severe and often include *acting out* (q.v.) and behavior suggesting *schizophrenia* (q.v.).

brain syndrome: An organic psychiatric disorder characterized by impairment of orientation, memory, intellectual functions and judgment, together with emotional instability. The disability may be due to such factors as injury, aging, toxins, infections, or tumors. May be acute or chronic, reversible or irreversible.

brain waves: See *E.E.G.*

Brigham, Amariah (1798-1849): One of the original thirteen founders of the American Psychiatric Association and the founder and first editor of its official journal, the *American Journal of Psychiatry* (1844).

Brill, A. A. (1874-1948): Pupil of Freud; first American psychoanalyst. Noted for his translations of Freud's works.

bulimia: Morbidly increased hunger. Same as *polyphagia* (q.v.).

carbon dioxide therapy: See under *shock treatment.*

castration: In psychiatry, usually the fantasied loss of the penis. Also used figuratively to denote state of impotence, powerlessness, helplessness, or defeat, etc. See also *castration complex* under *complex.*

castration anxiety: Anxiety due to danger (fantasied) of loss of the genitals or injuries to them. May be precipitated by everyday events which have symbolic significance and appear to be threatening such as loss of job, loss of a tooth, or an experience of ridicule or humiliation. See also *castration complex* under *complex.*

castration complex: See under *complex.*

catalepsy: A generalized condition of diminished responsiveness usually characterized by trance-like states. May occur in organic or psychological disorders or under hypnosis.

cataplexy: Momentary loss of skeletal muscular tone with resulting weakness.

catatonic state (catatonia): A state characterized by immobility with muscular rigidity or inflexibility and at times by excitability. Virtually always a symptom of *schizophrenia.*

catecholamines: A group of *biogenic amines* derived from phenylalanine and containing the catechol nucleus. Certain of these amines, such as *epinephrine* and *norepinephrine* exert an important influence on nervous system activity.

catharsis: (1) The healthful (therapeutic) release of ideas through a "talking out" of conscious material accompanied by the appropriate emotional reaction. (2) The release into awareness of repressed (i.e. "forgotten") material from the unconscious. Catharsis and *abreaction* (q.v.) are sometimes incorrectly used interchangeably.

cathexis: Attachment, conscious or unconscious, of emotional feeling and significance to an idea or object, most commonly a person.

causalgia: A sensation of burning pain of either organic or psychic origin.

censor: In psychoanalytic theory, a part of the unconscious self (i.e. the superego and parts of the ego) which functions as a guard, as in dreams, to prevent the emergence of repressed material into consciousness.

central nervous system (CNS): The brain and spinal cord.

cephalalgia: Headache or head pain.

cerea flexibilitas: The "waxy flexibility" often present in catatonic schizophrenia in which the patient's arm or leg remains passively in the position in which it is placed.

character: In psychiatry, the sum of the relatively fixed personality traits and habitual modes of response of an individual.

character analysis: Psychoanalytic treatment aimed at the *character defenses.*

character defense: The concept that character or personality traits serve an unconscious defensive purpose. See also *character disorder.*

character disorder: A syndrome characterized by unhealthy patterns of behavior and emotional responses such as *acting out* (q.v.) which are to varying degrees socially unacceptable or disapproved. There is usually very little evidence of anxiety or symptoms as ordinarily seen in the neuroses. The symptoms are *ego-syntonic* (q.v.). Approximates concept of *character neurosis.*

character neurosis: Similar to *character disorder* except that the neurotic conflicts are expressed in exaggerated but socially acceptable patterns of behavior and may not be easily recognizable as symptoms.

child analysis: Application of modified psychoanalytic methods and goals to problems of children to remove impediments to normal personality development.

childhood schizophrenia: A loosely used term, usually indicating a wide variety of psychotic-like manifestations in children which may be secondary to organic processes or primary

ary with multiple etiologies. Its symptoms often include *autism*.

cholinergic: Activated or transmitted by acetylcholine (e.g. *parasympathetic nerve fibers*). See also *parasympathetic nervous system*.

claustrophobia: See *phobia*.

climacteric: Menopausal period in women. Also used sometimes to refer to the corresponding age period in men.

clinical psychologist: See *psychologist, clinical*.

cognitive: Refers to the mental processes of comprehension, judgment, memory, and reasoning, as opposed to emotional and volitional processes.

collective unconscious: In Jungian theory a portion of the unconscious common to all mankind; also called racial unconscious. See *unconscious, Jung*.

combat fatigue: Disabling physical and emotional fatigue incident to military combat; also used during World War II as a synonym for combat neurosis.

commitment: In psychiatry, the legal process for the mandatory hospitalization of an individual in need of treatment for a mental disorder. To be distinguished from medical, informal, voluntary, and other forms of admission to a hospital.

community mental health center: A community-based facility, or a complex of such facilities, for the prevention and treatment of mental illness. May include a full spectrum of services such as inpatient, outpatient, day hospital, night hospital, emergency, aftercare, rehabilitation, public education, consultation, and evaluation services. See also *community psychiatry*.

community psychiatry: A broad and relatively recent term referring to the use of all available forces, resources and techniques that facilitate the treatment of the psychiatric patient in his own community.

compensation: (1) A defense mechanism, operating unconsciously, by which the individual attempts to make up for (i.e. to compensate for) real or fancied deficiencies. (2) A conscious process in which the individual strives to make up for real or imagined defects in such areas as physique, performance, skills, or psychological attributes. The two types frequently merge.

compensation neurosis: Certain neurotic reactions in which features of secondary gain (e.g. situational or financial) are prominent. See *secondary gain*.

complex: A group of associated ideas which have a common strong emotional tone. These are largely unconscious, and significantly influence attitudes and associations. Three examples are:

castration complex: A group of emotionally charged ideas which are unconscious, and which refer to the fear of losing the genital organs, usually as punishment for forbidden sexual desires. Includes the childhood fantasy that female genitals result from loss of a penis.

inferiority complex (Adler): Feelings of inferiority stemming from real or imagined physical or social inadequacies which may cause anxiety or other adverse reactions. The individual may overcompensate by excessive ambition or by the development of special skills, often in the very field in which he was originally handicapped. See also *overcompensation*.

oedipus complex (Freud): Attachment of the child for the parent of the opposite sex, accompanied by envious and aggressive feelings toward the parent of the same sex. These feelings are largely repressed (i.e. made unconscious) because of the fear of displeasure or punishment by the parent of the same sex. In its original use, the term applied only to the male child.

compulsion: An insistent, repetitive, intrusive, and unwanted urge to perform an act which is contrary to the person's ordinary conscious wishes or standards. A defensive substitute for hidden and still more unacceptable ideas and wishes. Failure to perform the compulsive act results in overt anxiety.

compulsive personality: A personality characterized by excessive adherence to rigid standards. Typically, the individual is inflexible, overconscientious, overinhibited, unable to relax, and exhibits repetitive patterns of behavior.

compulsive ritual: Series of acts repetitively carried out under compulsion. As with single compulsions, failure to carry out the ritual results in tension and anxiety.

conative: Pertains to the basic strivings of an individual, as expressed in his behavior and actions, volitional as opposed to cognitive.

ondensation: A psychologic process often present in dreams
n which two or more concepts are fused so that a single
ymbol represents the multiple components.

onditioned reflex (CR): A reflex developed by repetitive
xperience in association with another stimulus. E.g., a dog
s repeatedly offered food while a bell is rung. After a period
he ringing of the bell alone will bring on salivation. The con-
itioned stimulus (the bell) is the signal for the conditioned
eflex (salivation); the unconditioned stimulus (food) is the
dequate physiological stimulus for the *unconditioned reflex,
UCR* (q.v.).

onfabulation: The more or less unconscious, defensive "fill-
ng in" of actual memory gaps by imaginary experiences,
often complex, that are recounted in a detailed and plausible
vay. Seen principally in organic psychotic reactions, such as
Korsakoff's psychosis (q.v.).

onflict: The clash, largely determined by unconscious fac-
ors, between two opposing emotional forces. For example, an
nstinctual wish for gratification may conflict with restric-
ions of conscience (intrapsychic conflict), or with external
social requirements. Conflict is basic in psychic life and
undamental in the etiology of psychological disorders.

> **extra-psychic conflict:** Conflict between the self and the
> environment.

> **intra-psychic conflict:** Conflict within the personality.

confusion: Disturbed orientation in respect to time, place,
or person; sometimes accompanied by disturbances of consciousness.

congenital: Present at birth.

conscience: The morally self-critical part of oneself wherein
have developed and reside standards of behavior, performance, and value judgments. Commonly equated with the conscious *superego* (q.v.).

constitution: A person's intrinsic physical and psychological
endowment; sometimes used more narrowly to indicate the
physical inheritance or potential from birth.

constitutional types: Constellations of morphological, physiological, and psychologic traits as earlier proposed by various

21

scholars. Galen, Kretschmer, and Sheldon proposed the following major types: *Galen:* sanguine, melancholic, choleric and phlegmatic types; *Kretschmer:* pyknic (stocky), asthenic (slender), athletic, and dysplastic (disproportioned) types; *Sheldon:* ectomorphic, mesomorphic, and endomorphic types based on the relative preponderance of outer, middle or inner layers of embryonic cellular tissue.

constructive aggression: See under *aggression*.

conversion: A mental mechanism, operating unconsciously, by which intrapsychic conflicts, which would otherwise give rise to anxiety, are instead given symbolic external expression. The repressed ideas or impulses, plus the psychologic defenses against them, are converted into a variety of somatic symptoms. Example: psychogenic paralysis of a limb which prevents its use for aggressive purposes.

conversion reaction: See under *psychoneurosis*.

convulsive disorders: Primarily grand mal, petit-mal, Jacksonian, and psychomotor epilepsy. May occur in any organic cerebral disease. See *epilepsy*.

coprophagia: Eating of filth or feces.

coprophilia: Excessive or morbid interest in filth or feces or symbolic representations thereof.

countertransference: The psychiatrist's conscious or unconscious emotional reaction to his patient. See also *transference*.

cretinism: Severe thyroid deficiency, usually accompanied by mental deficiency and bodily malformation.

criminally insane: A legal term for patients who have been committed to a mental hospital by the courts after being found not guilty of a crime "by reason of insanity."

cunnilingus: Sexual activity in which the mouth and tongue are used to stimulate the female genitals.

cybernetics: Term introduced by Norbert Wiener (1894-1964) to designate the science of control mechanisms. It covers the entire field of communication and control in machines and puts forth the hypothesis that there is some similarity between the human nervous system and electronic control devices.

cyclothymic personality: A personality characterized by alternating moods of elation and sadness with mood swings out

f proportion to apparent stimuli. The moods result from in-
ernal causes rather than from external events. In severe
orm, *manic-depressive psychosis.*

day hospital: A special facility or an arrangement within a
hospital setting which enables the patient to come to the hospital for treatment during the day and return home at night.
See also *night hospital.*

death instinct (Thanatos): In Freudian theory, the unconscious drive toward dissolution and death. Coexists with and
is in opposition to the life instinct *Eros.*

defense mechanism: Specific intrapsychic defensive processes, operating unconsciously, which are employed to seek
relief from emotional conflict and freedom from anxiety.
Conscious efforts are frequently made for the same reasons,
but true defense mechanisms are out of awareness (unconscious). Some of the common defense mechanisms defined in
this Glossary are: *compensation, conversion, denial, displacement, dissociation, idealization, identification, incorporation, introjection, projection, rationalization, reaction formation, regression, repression, sublimation, substitution, symbolization, undoing.* See also *mental mechanism.*

déjà vu: A subjective feeling that an experience which is occurring for the first time has been experienced before.

delirium: A mental state characterized by disorientation and
confusion. Anxiety, fear, illusions, or hallucinations may also
be present. Examples: The delirium of fever, delirium tre-
mens (alcoholic), bromide intoxication.

delusion: A false belief out of keeping with the individual level of knowledge and his cultural group. The belief results from unconscious needs and is maintained against logical argument and despite objective contradictory evidence. Common delusions include:

delusions of grandeur: Exaggerated ideas of one's importance or identity.

delusions of persecution: Ideas that one has been singled out for persecution. See also *paranoia*.

delusions of reference: Incorrect assumption that certain casual or unrelated remarks or the behavior of others apply to oneself. See also *paranoia*.

dementia: An old term denoting madness or insanity; now used entirely to denote organic loss of intellectual function.

dementia praecox: Obsolescent descriptive term for *schizophrenia*. Introduced by Morel (1860) and later popularized by *Kraepelin* (q.v.).

dementia, senile: A chronic brain disorder caused by a generalized atrophy of the brain due to aging. See *senile psychosis*.

denial: A defense mechanism, operating unconsciously, used to resolve emotional conflict and allay anxiety by denying a thought, feeling, wish, need or external reality factor which is consciously intolerable.

dependency needs: Vital infantile needs for mothering, love, affection, shelter, protection, security, food, and warmth. May continue beyond infancy in overt or hidden forms, or may be increased in the adult as a regressive manifestation.

depersonalization: Feelings of unreality or strangeness concerning either the environment or the self or both.

depressed phase: See under *manic depressive reactions*.

depression: Psychiatrically, a morbid sadness, dejection, or melancholy; to be differentiated from grief, which is realistic and proportionate to what has been lost. A depression may be a symptom of any psychiatric disorder or may constitute its principal manifestation. Neurotic depressions are differentiated from psychotic depressions in that they do not involve loss of capacity for *reality testing*. The major psychotic deressions include *agitated depression, involutional psychosis,* and the depressed phase of *manic-depressive psychosis.*

epressive reaction: See under *psychoneurosis.*

eprivation, emotional: A lack of adequate and appropriate terpersonal and/or environmental experience, usually in the arly developmental years.

eprivation, sensory: Term for experience of being cut off om external sensory stimuli and the opportunity for perception. May occur accidentally (e.g. a marooned explorer) r experimentally. May lead to disorganized thinking, depression, panic, delusion formation, and/or hallucinations.

epth psychology: The psychology of unconscious mental rocesses. Also a system of psychology in which the study of uch processes plays a major role, as in *psychoanalysis* (q.v.).

ereistic: Describes mental activity that is not in accordance vith reality, logic, or experience. Similar to autistic. See *utism.*

escriptive psychiatry: A system of psychiatry based upon bservation and study of readily observable external factors; o be differentiated from dynamic psychiatry. Often used to efer to the systematized descriptions of mental illnesses formulated by *Kraepelin* (q.v.). See also *dynamic psychiatry; psychiatry.*

desoxyribonucleic acid: See *DNA.*

destructive aggression: See under *aggression.*

deterioration: In psychiatry, the progressive disintegration of intellectual and/or emotional functions. May or may not be reversible.

determinism: A doctrine common to all sciences. In psychiatry, it postulates that nothing in the individual's emotional or mental life results from chance alone but rather from specific causes or forces known or unknown.

dipsomania: See *mania.*

disorientation: Loss of awareness of the position of the self in relation to space, time, or other persons.

displacement: A defense mechanism, operating unconsciously, in which an emotion is transferred or "displaced" from its original object to a more acceptable substitute.

dissociation: A psychologic separation or splitting off; a intrapsychic defensive process which operates automaticall and unconsciously. Through its operation, emotional signif cance and affect are separated and detached from an ide situation, or object. Dissociation may, unconsciously, def or postpone experiencing the emotional impact as, for examp in selective amnesia. Also a *mental mechanism* (q.v.), an often a *defense mechanism* (q.v.).

dissociative reaction: See under *psychoneurosis*.

distortion: In Freudian theory, a prime mechanism which, i dreams, together with *condensation* (q.v.), *symbolizatio* (q.v.), and *overdetermination* (q.v.) aids in the repression an disguise of unacceptable thoughts. See also *mental mechanism*

parataxic distortion: Sullivan's term for certain distortio in judgment and perception, particularly in interpersona relations, based upon the observer's need to perceive sul jects and relationships in accordance with a pattern set b earlier experience. Parataxic distortions develop as a de fense against anxiety. See *Sullivan*.

distributive analysis and synthesis: The therapy used b the psychobiologic school of psychiatry developed by Ado Meyer. Entails extensive guided and directed investigatio and analysis of the patient's entire past experience, stressin his assets and liabilities to make possible a constructive syr thesis. See *psychobiology, Meyer*.

Dix, Dorothea Lynde (1802-1887): American pioneer in th crusade to improve institutional care of the mentally ill.

DNA (desoxyribonucleic acid): One of the key chemical governing life functions. Found in the cell nucleus. Essenti constituent of the genes. Governs the manufacture of *RN* (q.v.) and certain other proteins.

Don Juan: Legendary seducer and "lover." In psychiatry, de notes compulsive or anxiety-driven sexual overactivity i males.

double personality: See *personality, multiple*.

Down's syndrome: See *mongolism*.

drive: Basic urge, instinct, motivation. In psychiatry, a term currently preferred to avoid confusion with the more purel biological concept of *instinct* (q.v.).

dummy: See *placebo*.

Durham decision: Refers to a decision by the U.S. Court of Appeals for the District of Columbia (1954) in which the Court stated that the *McNaghten Rule* and the *Irresistible Impulse Test* were not consonant with the realities of mental life as reflected in modern psychiatry and held that "an accused is not criminally responsible if his unlawful act was the product of mental disease or mental defect." (Durham v. U.S., 214 F 2d 862). Under the Durham test, a psychiatrist may give any relevant testimony about the mental illness at issue, whereas before his testimony had been confined to a determination of whether the accused could distinguish between "right and wrong" or acted under an "irresistible impulse." The Durham test proceeds on the assumption that when the criminal act of the accused is the product of his mental illness, the suggested conclusion is that the accused should be hospitalized for treatment and possible rehabilitation, a premise more in harmony with modern psychiatric thought than the earlier tests of legal responsibility.

dyadic: The relationship between a pair. In psychiatry, refers to the therapeutic relationship between doctor and patient as in "dyadic therapy."

dynamic psychiatry: As distinguished from *descriptive psychiatry,* refers to the study of emotional processes, their origins, and the mental mechanisms. Implies the study of the active, energy-laden, and changing factors in human behavior and its motivation, as opposed to the older, more static and descriptive study of clinical patterns, symptoms, and classification. Dynamic principles convey the concepts of change, of evolution, and progression or regression.

dynamics: Refers to emotional forces which determine the pattern of feelings and behavior. These forces arise through the interaction of *drives* and defenses in growth and development.

dynamism: See *mental mechanism*.

dysarthria: Impaired, difficult speech, usually due to organic disorders of the nervous system or speech organs.

dyspareunia: Pelvic pain, usually emotional in origin. Experienced by the female in sexual intercourse.

dysphagia: Difficult or painful swallowing.

early infantile autism (Kanner's syndrome): See under *autism.*

echolalia: The pathological repetition by some psychotic patients of phrases or words said in their presence. Most frequent in certain schizophrenic disorders.

echopraxia: Pathological repetition by some psychotic patients of movements made by another person in their presence.

ecology, human: The branch of science dealing with the interaction of the human organism with its total environment.

E.C.T. (electroconvulsive therapy): See under *shock treatment.*

E.E.G. (brain waves): Electroencephalogram. A graphic recording of minute electrical impulses arising from activity of cells in the brain. Used in neurologic and psychiatric diagnosis and research.

ego: In psychoanalytic theory, one of the three major divisions in the model of the psychic apparatus, the others being the *id* and *superego.* The ego represents the sum of certain *mental mechanisms,* such as perception and memory, and specific defensive mechanisms. The ego serves to mediate between the demands of primitive instinctual drives (the id), or internalized parental and social prohibitions (the superego) and of reality. The compromises between these forces achieved by the ego tend to resolve intrapsychic conflict and serve an adaptive and executive function. As used in psychiatry, the term should not be confused with its common usage in the sense of "self-love" or "selfishness."

ego analysis: Intensive psychoanalytic study and analysis of the ways in which the ego resolves or attempts to deal with intrapsychic conflicts, especially in relation to the development of mental mechanisms and the maturation of capacity for rational thought and action. Modern psychoanalysis gives

28

more emphasis to considerations of the defensive operations of the ego than did earlier techniques which emphasized instinctual forces to a greater degree.

ego-dystonic: At variance with or repugnant to the ego.

ego ideal: That part of the personality which comprises the aims and goals of the self; usually refers to the conscious or unconscious emulation of significant figures with whom the person has identified. The ego ideal emphasizes what one should be or do in contrast to what one should not be or do.

ego instincts: In Freudian theory before 1921, the ego instincts referred to self-preservative needs and self-love as opposed to object love (i.e., love of another person), in opposition to the libidinal instinct. Though obsolescent, the term is sometimes used for drives which are primarily erotic, such as for power, prestige, acquisition, or self-preservation.

egomania: See under *mania.*

ego-syntonic: Acceptable to or consonant with the aims of the *ego.*

eidetic image: Unusually vivid and apparently exact mental image; may be a memory, fantasy, or dream.

elaboration: An unconscious psychologic process of expansion and embellishment of detail, especially with reference to a symbol or representation in a dream.

Electra complex: Obsolescent term. Analogous in the female to *oedipus complex* (q.v. under *complex).*

electroconvulsive treatment (E.C.T.): See under *shock treatment.*

electroencephalogram: See *E.E.G.*

electroshock therapy (E.C.T. or E.S.T.): See under *shock treatment.*

electro-stimulation: See under *shock treatment.*

elope (elopement): In hospital psychiatry, a term sometimes used for a patient who leaves a mental hospital without permission. See also *parole, escape.*

emotion: A feeling such as fear, anger, grief, joy, or love. As used in psychiatry, the patient may not always be conscious of the feeling. Synonymous with *affect.*

emotional deprivation: See *deprivation, emotional.*

emotionally disturbed: Often used to describe a person with a *mental disorder* (q.v.).

emotional health: See *mental health.*

emotional illness: Often used synonymously with *mental disorder* (q.v.).

empathy: An objective and insightful awareness of the feelings, emotions and behavior of another person, their meaning and significance. To be distinguished from sympathy, which is usually nonobjective and noncritical.

engram: A memory trace. Theoretically, a protoplasmic change in neural tissue to explain persistence of memory.

entropy: Diminished capacity for spontaneous change such as occurs in aging.

enuresis: Bed-wetting.

epilepsy: A disorder characterized by periodic motor or sensory seizures or their equivalents, and sometimes accompanied by a loss of consciousness, or by certain equivalent manifestations. May be idiopathic (no known organic cause) or symptomatic (due to organic lesions). Usually accompanied by abnormal electrical discharge as shown by *E.E.G.* (q.v.).

> **epileptic equivalent:** Episodic, sensory, motor, or experiential phenomena that may replace convulsive seizures in epilepsy.

> **Jacksonian epilepsy:** Recurrent episodes of localized convulsive seizures or spasms limited to a part or region of the body, without loss of consciousness. Named after Hughlings Jackson (1835-1911).

> **major epilepsy (grand mal):** Characterized by gross convulsive seizures, with loss of consciousness.

> **minor epilepsy (petit mal):** Minor nonconvulsive epileptic seizures or equivalents; may be limited to only momentary lapses of consciousness.

> **psychomotor epilepsy:** Recurrent periodic disturbances, usually of behavior, during which the patient carries out movement often repetitive, highly organized but semiautomatic in character.

epileptic equivalent: See under *epilepsy.*

epinephrine: One of the *catecholamines* (q.v.). Secreted by the adrenal glands. Also known as adrenalin.

erogenous zone: See *erotogenic zone*.

erotic: Consciously or unconsciously invested with sexual feeling; sensually related.

erotogenic zone: An area of the body particularly susceptible to erotic arousal when stimulated, and especially the oral, anal, and genital areas, more diffuse in infancy. Sometimes called *erogenous zone*.

erotomania: See *mania*.

escape (escapee): In psychiatry, the departure of a patient from a mental hospital without permission. Inappropriately used except with reference to a patient confined in the *maximum security unit* of a mental hospital by court order. See also *elope*.

E.S.P.: See *extra-sensory perception*.

E.S.T. (also E.C.T.): See *electroshock therapy*.

ethology: A systematic study of comparative animal behavior.

etiology: Causation, particularly with reference to disease.

euphoria: An exaggerated feeling of physical and emotional well-being not consonant with apparent stimuli or events; usually of psychologic origin, but also seen in organic brain disease and toxic states.

executant ego function: A term for the ego's management of the *mental mechanisms* in order to meet the needs of the organism.

exhibitionism: Commonly, "showing off." Psychiatrically, body exposure, usually of the male genitals to females. Sexual stimulation or gratification usually accompanies the act.

existential psychiatry: A school of psychiatry based on the existential philosophy of Kierkegaard, Sartre, and others.

extrapsychic conflict: See under *conflict*.

extrapyramidal syndrome: A pathological condition which may occur as a side effect of certain *psychotropic* drugs. Usually characterized by muscular rigidity, tremors, and sometimes peculiar involuntary movements or postures. Parkinson's disease is basically the same syndrome when caused by chronic lesions in the brain.

extrapyramidal system: That portion of the brain concerned with nonvoluntary, skeletal, muscular control.

extrasensory perception (E.S.P.): That which is apparently known or perceived without recourse to the conventional use of any of the physical senses.

extroversion: A state in which attention and energies are largely directed outward from the self, as opposed to interest primarily directed toward the self as in *introversion*. (Spelled *extraversion* by Jung).

fantasy: An imagined sequence of events or mental images, e.g., day dreams. Serves to express unconscious conflicts or to gratify unconscious wishes.

fear: Normal emotional response to consciously recognized and external sources of danger, to be distinguished from anxiety. See *anxiety; phobia.*

feeblemindedness: Obsolete. See *mental retardation.*

fellatio: Sexual stimulation of the penis by oral contact.

fetish: An inanimate object, such as an article of apparel, symbolically endowed with special meaning. Often necessary for completion of the sexual act.

fetishism: Process of attachment of special meaning to an inanimate object (or fetish) which serves, usually unconsciously, as a substitute for the original object or person. The substitute object is often a neurotic source of sexual stimulation or gratification.

fixation: The arrest of psychosexual maturation. Depending on degree it may be either normal or pathologic. See *psychosexual development.*

flagellantism: A masochistic or sadistic act in which one or both participants derive stimulation, usually erotic, from whipping or being whipped.

flexibilitas cerea: See *cerea flexibilitas.*

flight of ideas: Verbal skipping from one idea to another before the last one has been concluded; the ideas appear to be continuous, but are fragmentary and determined by chance associations. Sometimes seen in the manic phase of *manic depressive reaction* (q.v.) and *schizophrenia.*

folie à deux: A psychotic reaction in which two closely related persons, usually in the same family, mutually share the same delusions.

forensic psychiatry: That branch of psychiatry dealing with the legal aspects of mental disorders.

forepleasure: Sexual play preceding intercourse.

formication: In psychiatry, the tactile hallucination that insects are crawling on the body.

free association: In psychoanalytic therapy, spontaneous, uncensored verbalization by the patient of whatever comes to mind.

free floating anxiety: Severe, generalized, persisting *anxiety.* Often a precursor of *panic.*

Freud, Sigmund (1856-1939): Founder of *psychoanalysis.* Most of the basic concepts of dynamic psychiatry are derived from his theories.

frigidity: The female's inability to respond adequately and fully to sexual intercourse.

fugue: A major state of personality dissociation characterized by amnesia and actual physical flight from the immediate environment.

functional illness: An illness of emotional origin in which organic or structural changes are either absent or develop secondarily to prolonged emotional stress.

g

Ganser syndrome: Sometimes called "nonsense syndrome" or "syndrome of approximate answers" (e.g. "two times two equals about ten"). Commonly used to characterize behavior of prisoners who seek to mislead others regarding their mental state.

general paresis: A psychosis associated with organic disease of the brain resulting from chronic syphilitic infection.

geriatrics: A branch of medicine dealing with the processes and diseases of the aging.

Gestalt psychology: A German school of psychology which places emphasis on a total perceptual configuration and the interrelations of its component parts.

globus hystericus: An hysterical symptom in which there is a disturbing sensation of a lump in the throat. See also *conversion reaction* under *psychoneurosis*.

grand mal: See *epilepsy*.

grandiose: In psychiatry, refers to delusions of great wealth, power or fame.

grief: Normal, appropriate emotional response to an external and consciously recognized loss; self-limiting, and gradually subsiding within a reasonable time. To be distinguished from *depression* (q.v.).

gross stress reaction: A diagnostic term employed for certain acute emotional reactions incident to severe environmental stress as, for example, in military operations, industrial, domestic, or civilian disasters, and other life situations.

group psychotherapy: Application of psychotherapeutic techniques to a group including utilization of interactions of members of the group.

h

halfway house: In psychiatry, a specialized residence for mental patients who do not require full hospitalization but who need an intermediate degree of protection and support before returning to fully independent community living.

hallucination: A false sensory perception in the absence of an actual external stimulus. May be induced by emotional and/or such other factors as drugs, alcohol, and stress. May occur in any of the senses.

hallucinogen: A chemical agent that produces hallucinations

hallucinosis: A state in which the patient is constantly hallucinated. Example: chronic alcoholic hallucinosis.

hebephrenia: See *schizophrenia.*

hedonism: In psychiatry, constant seeking of pleasure and avoidance of pain. Often seen in *character disorders.* See also *anhedonia.*

hermaphrodite: An individual who possesses both male and female sexual organs to some degree. Almost invariably one sex is predominant.

homeostasis: The maintenance of self-regulating metabolic or psychologic processes which are optimal for comfort and survival.

homosexual panic: An acute and severe attack of anxiety based upon unconscious conflicts involving homosexuality.

homosexuality: Sexual attraction or relationship between members of the same sex.

overt homosexuality: Homosexuality which is consciously recognized or practiced.

latent homosexuality: A condition characterized by unconscious homosexual desires.

Horney, Karen (1885-1952): Psychiatrist and psychoanalyst. She proposed a theory of neurosis based on an optimistic philosophy of human nature which emphasized the urge toward self-realization and stressed environmental and cultural factors.

Huntington's chorea: An uncommon and progressively degenerative disease occurring in families. Onset is in adult life. Characterized by random movements (lurching, jerking) of the entire body and progressive mental deterioration.

hyperkinesis: Increased or excessive muscular activity seen in some neurological conditions, but more frequently in psychiatric disorders, especially in children.

hyperkinetic: Describes a state of muscular overactivity.

hypesthesia: A state of diminished sensitivity to tactile stimuli.

hypnagogic: Produced or induced by sleep or related states. *Hypnagogic imagery* refers to the mental images that may occur just before sleep.

hypnagogic hallucinations: Hallucinations occurring during the hypnagogic state. Usually of no pathologic significance.

hypnosis: A state of increased receptivity to suggestion and direction, initially induced by the influence of another person. Often characterized by an altered state of consciousness, similar to that observed in spontaneous dissociative conditions. The degree may vary from mild hypersuggestibility to a trance state with complete surgical anesthesia.

hypochondriasis: Persistent overconcern with the state of physical or emotional health accompanied by various bodily complaints without demonstrable organic pathology.

hypomania: A mild form of manic activity. See also *manic depressive reaction.*

hysteria: An illness resulting from emotional conflict and generally characterized by immaturity, impulsiveness, attention-seeking, dependency, and the use of the defense mechanisms of conversion and dissociation. Classically manifested by dramatic physical symptoms involving the voluntary muscles or the organs of special senses. See also *conversion and dissociative reactions* under *psychoneurosis.*

hysterical personality: A personality type characterized by shifting emotional feelings, susceptibility to suggestion, impulsive behavior, attention-seeking, immaturity, and self-absorption; not necessarily disabling.

hysterics: Lay term for uncontrollable emotional outbursts.

iatrogenic illness: An emotional illness unwittingly precipitated or induced by the physician's attitude, examination, or comments.

id: In Freudian theory, that part of the personality structure which harbors the unconscious instinctive desires and strivings of the individual. See also *ego, superego.*

idealization: A defense mechanism, operating consciously or unconsciously, in which there is overestimation of some admired aspect or attribute of another person.

ideas of reference: Incorrect interpretation of casual incidents and external events as having direct reference to one's self. May reach sufficient intensity to constitute *delusions.*

idée fixe: Fixed idea. Loosely used to describe a compulsive drive, an obsessive idea, or a delusion.

identification: A defense mechanism, operating unconsciously, by which an individual endeavors to pattern himself after another. Identification plays a major role in the development of one's personality and specifically of one's superego, including the conscience. To be differentiated from imitation as a conscious process.

idiopathic: Of unknown cause.

idiot: Obsolescent term. See *mental retardation.*

idiot-savant: An individual with gross mental retardation who nonetheless is capable of performing certain remarkable "intellectual" feats such as calendar calculation and puzzle solving.

illusion: The misinterpretation of a real, external sensory experience.

imago: In Jungian psychology, an unconscious mental image, usually idealized, of an important person in the early history of the individual.

imbecile: Obsolescent term. See *mental retardation.*

impotence: Usually refers to inability of the male to perform the sexual act, generally for psychologic reasons; more broadly used to indicate lack of sexual vigor, powerlessness.

imprinting: A relatively recent term used in *ethology* (q.v.) to refer to the process of rapid learning and behavioral patterning which occurs at critical points in very early stages of development in animals and which is based on adult models. The degree to which imprinting applies to human learning has not been established.

impulse: A psychic striving; usually refers to an instinctive urge.

incompetent: A legal term for a person who, because of mental defect, cannot be held responsible in certain legal procedures such as making a will, entering into a contract, or standing trial.

incorporation: A primitive defense mechanism, operating unconsciously, in which the psychic representation of a person, or parts of him, are figuratively ingested. Example: infantile fantasy that the mother's breast has been ingested and is part of one's self.

individual psychology: The system of psychiatric theory, research, and therapy developed by Alfred Adler which stresses *compensation* and *overcompensation* (q.v.) for inferiority feelings. See also *Adler.*

industrial psychiatry: See *occupational psychiatry.*

inferiority complex: See *complex.*

inhibition: Interference with or restriction of specific activities; the result of an unconscious defense against forbidden instinctual drives.

insanity: Vague, legal term for the psychotic state, now obsolete in psychiatric usage. Generally connotes: (a) a mental incompetence, (b) inability to distinguish "right from wrong," and/or (c) a condition which interferes with the individual's ability to care for himself or which constitutes a danger to himself or to others. See *McNaghten Rule; Durham Decision.*

insight: Self-understanding. A major goal of psychotherapy. The extent of the individual's understanding of the origin, nature, and mechanisms of his attitudes and behavior. More superficially, recognition by a patient that he is mentally ill.

instinct: An inborn *drive* (q.v.). The human instincts include those of self-preservation, sexuality, and (for some authors), aggression, the *ego instincts* (q.v.) and the herd or social instincts. See also *death instinct*.

insulin treatment: See *shock treatment*.

integration: The useful organization and incorporation of both new and old data, experience, and emotional capacities into the personality. Also refers to the organization and amalgamation of functions at various levels of *psychosexual development* (q.v.).

intellectualization: The defense mechanism which utilizes reasoning as a defense against conscious confrontation with the unconscious conflict and its stressful emotions.

intelligence: The potential ability of an individual to understand what he needs to recall and to mobilize and integrate constructively previous learning and experience in meeting new situations. The ability to use intelligence is influenced by emotional factors.

intelligence quotient (IQ): A numerical rating determined through psychological testing which indicates approximately the relationship of a person's mental age (MA) to his chronological age (CA). Expressed mathematically as $IQ = MA/CA$ x100. Thus, if $MA = 6$ and $CA = 12$, then $IQ = 6/12$x100 or 50 (retarded). If $MA = 12$ and $CA = 12$, then $IQ = 100$ (average). If $MA = 18$ and $CA = 12$, then $IQ = 150$ (very superior). (Note: Since intellectual capacity is assumed to be fully developed between the ages of 15 and 16, adult IQs are computed by using a fixed arbitrary value of 15 for CA.)

interpretation: The process by which the therapist communicates to the patient understanding of a particular aspect of his problems or behavior.

intrapsychic: That which takes place within the *psyche* or mind.

intrapsychic conflict: See under *conflict*.

introjection: A defense mechanism, operating unconsciously, whereby loved or hated external objects are taken within oneself symbolically. The converse of *projection* (q.v.). May serve as a defense against conscious recognition of intolerable hostile impulses. For example, in severe depression, the individual may unconsciously direct unacceptable hatred or aggression toward himself, i.e., toward the introjected object within himself. Related to the more primitive mechanism of *incorporation* (q.v.).

introversion: Preoccupation with oneself, with accompanying reduction of interest in the outside world. Roughly the reverse of *extroversion* (q.v.).

involutional psychosis (involutional melancholia): A psychotic reaction occurring in late middle life. Formerly thought to be related to the menopause in the female and the climacteric in the male. Characterized most commonly by depression and occasionally paranoid thinking. The course tends to be prolonged and the condition may be manifested by feelings of guilt, anxiety, agitation, severe insomnia, and somatic preoccupations, often of a delusional or nihilistic nature.

inward aggression: See under *aggression*.

I.Q.: See *intelligence quotient*.

irresistible impulse test: A test for determining criminal responsibility. The District of Columbia courts in 1929 (Smith v. U.S., 36 F 2nd 548, 549) supplemented the McNaghten "right or wrong" test by holding that the accused could not be held criminally responsible if it could be demonstrated that he was impelled to commit the act by an irresistible impulse. The assumption here was that the mental illness produces sudden or spontaneous impulses to commit unlawful acts. See also *McNaghten Rule; Durham decision*.

isolation: An unconscious defense mechanism in which an unacceptable impulse, idea, or act is separated from its original memory source thereby removing the emotional charge associated with the original memory.

j

Jacksonian epilepsy: See *epilepsy*.

Janet, Pierre (1859-1947): French psychiatrist. Described *psychasthenia* (q.v.) which is sometimes referred to as Janet's disease. Also first to use term la *belle indifférence* (q.v.).

Joint Commission on Mental Illness and Health: A multidisciplinary agency, incorporated in 1956, and representing thirty-six national agencies in the mental health and welfare fields. It conducted a five-year study of the mental health needs of the nation between 1956 and 1961 as authorized by the Congress in the Mental Health Study Act of 1955. The final report of the Joint Commission, *Action for Mental Health,* led ultimately to legislation by the Congress in 1964 authorizing and appropriating funds to facilitate the development of community mental health centers for the mentally ill and mentally retarded in the several states.

Jones, Ernest (1879-1958): Early pupil of Freud and his principal biographer. He pioneered in introducing psychoanalysis to the English-speaking world.

Jung, Carl Gustav (1875-1961): Swiss psychoanalyst. Founder of the school of *analytic psychology*.

Kirkbride, Thomas S. (1809-1883): American psychiatrist; one of the founders of the American Psychiatric Association. Noted for his pioneer contributions to mental hospital design.

kleptomania: See *mania.*

Korsakoff's psychosis: A mental disorder with brain damage characterized by amnesia, compensatory *confabulation* (q.v.), disturbance of attention and peripheral neuritis. Usually associated with alcoholism and dietary deficiencies.

Kraepelin, Emil (1865-1926): A German psychiatrist who developed an extensive systematic classification of mental diseases. See also *descriptive psychiatry.*

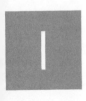

labile: Pertaining to rapidly shifting emotions; unstable.

lapsus linguae: A slip of the tongue due to unconscious factors.

latency period: In psychoanalytic theory, the phase between the oedipal period of psychosexual development (roughly 5-7 years) and the adolescent period. Characterized by an apparent cessation in psychosexual development.

latent content: The hidden (unconscious) meaning of thoughts or actions, especially in dreams or fantasies. In dreams it is expressed in distorted, disguised, condensed and symbolic form which is known as the *manifest content* (q.v.)

latent homosexuality: See under *homosexuality.*

lesbian: Homosexual woman.

libido: The psychic drive or energy usually associated with the sexual instinct. (Sexual is used here in the broad sense to include pleasure and love-object seeking.)

lobotomy: See *psychosurgery.*

logorrhea: Uncontrollable, excessive talking.

L. S. D. (lysergic acid diethylamide): A drug which produces symptoms and behavior resembling certain psychoses. These symptoms may include hallucinations, delusions, and time-space distortions.

lunacy: Obsolete legal term for a major mental illness.

lunatic: Obsolete legal term for a psychotic person.

m

magical thinking: A person's conviction that thinking equates with doing. Occurs in dreams, in children and primitive peoples, and in patients under a variety of conditions. Charcterized by lack of realistic relationship between cause and ffect.

aajor epilepsy (grand mal): See under *epilepsy.*

aalingering: A conscious simulation of illness used to avoid n unpleasant situation or for personal gain. In psychiatry, n indication of significant underlying pathology.

aania: A suffix denoting a pathological preoccupation with ome desire, idea or activity; a morbid compulsion. Some requently encountered manias are:

dipsomania: Compulsion to drink alcoholic beverages.

egomania: Pathological preoccupation with self.

erotomania: Pathological preoccupation with erotic fantasies or activities.

kleptomania: Compulsion to steal.

megalomania: Pathological preoccupation with delusions of power or wealth.

monomania: Pathological preoccupation with one subject.

necromania: Pathological preoccupation with dead bodies.

nymphomania: Abnormal and excessive need or desire for sexual intercourse in the female. Most nymphomaniacs, if not all, fail to achieve orgasm in the sexual act. See also *erotomania, Don Juan, satyriasis.*

pyromania: Morbid compulsion to set fires.

trichotillomania: Compulsion to pull out one's hair.

maniac: Imprecise, sensational, and misleading lay term for n emotionally disturbed person. Usually implies violent beavior. Is not specifically referable to any psychiatric diagnostic category.

manic depressive reaction: A group of psychiatric disorders marked by conspicuous mood swings ranging from normal to lation or to depression or alternating. Tendency to remission and recurrence. Officially regarded as a psychosis but may also exist in milder form.

depressed phase: Characterized by depression of mood with retardation and inhibition of thinking and physical activity. In some cases *agitation* may occur.

manic phase: Characterized by heightened excitability, a[c]celeration of thought, speech, and bodily motion, and [by] elation or grandiosity of mood and irritability.

manifest content: The remembered content of a dream [or] fantasy, as opposed to *latent content* which it conceals an[d] distorts.

MAO inhibitor (MAOI): Abbreviation for *monoamine oxidas[e] inhibitor* (q.v.).

masculine protest: Term coined by *Alfred Adler* to describ[e] a striving to escape identification with the feminine role. Ap[plies] primarily to women but may also be noted in the male[.] Adler regarded it as a main motive force in neurotic disease[.] It is characterized by aggressive behavior, masculine habit[s] and avoidance of traits presumably characteristic of th[e] female.

masochism: Pleasure derived from physical or psychologica[l] pain inflicted by oneself or by others. It may be conscious[ly] sought (flagellation in sexual perversions) or unconsciously a[r]ranged or invited. It carries the unconscious implication o[f] punishment for a sense of guilt in moral masochism. Thoug[h] sometimes obscure there is always a sexual component. Pres[ent] to some degree in all human relations and to greater de[grees] in all psychiatric disorders. It is the converse of *sadis[m]* (q.v.) and the two tend to coexist in the same individual.

maximum security unit: A prison-like building or ward with[in] in a mental hospital for confining and treating mental patient[s] who have committed crimes or whose symptoms are a phys[ical] ical threat to the safety of others. See also *criminally insane[.]*

McNaghten Rule (also M'Naghten, McNaughten): A lega[l] precedent in English law originating in 1843 (8 Eng. Rep. 718[)] in the trial of McNaghten for the murder of the Prime Min[ister's] ister's secretary. He was found not guilty, and the Englis[h] judges announced that the accused was not responsible fo[r] the crime if he was "labouring under such a defect of reason from disease of the mind, as not to know the nature and qual[ity] ity of the act he was doing; or, if he did know, that he di[d] not know he was doing what was wrong." This rule became known as the "right and wrong" test, and was widely adopted in the statutes of the English-speaking world. The rule did no[t] take account of the fact that a man might be held to be in

46

ane even though he knew the difference between right and wrong. See also *irresistible impulse test* and *Durham decision.*

megalomania: See *mania.*

melancholia: Severe depression, usually of psychotic depth. See *involutional psychosis.*

menarche: The beginning of menstrual functioning in the female life cycle.

mental age: The age level of mental ability determined by standard intelligence tests; distinguished from chronologic age.

mental deficiency: See *mental retardation.*

mental disease: See *mental disorder.*

mental disorder: Any psychiatric illness or disease included in the *Standard Nomenclature of Diseases and Operations* with the official approval of the American Medical Association. The same disorders are officially defined in the *Diagnostic and Statistical Manual for Mental Disorders,* published by the American Psychiatric Association (1952). Many of these disorders are described in this *Glossary.*

mental dynamism: Same as *mental mechanism* (q.v.).

mental health: A state of being which is relative rather than absolute, in which a person has effected a reasonably satisfactory integration of his instinctual drives. His integration is acceptable to himself and to his social milieu as reflected in his interpersonal relationships, his level of satisfaction in living, his actual achievement, his flexibility, and the level of maturity he has attained.

mental hygiene: A term used to designate measures employed to reduce the incidence of mental illness through prevention and early treatment and to promote mental health.

mental illness: Same as *mental disorder* (q.v.).

mental mechanism: A generic term for a variety of intrapsychic processes which are functions of the ego and largely unconscious. Includes perception, memory, thinking, and *defense mechanisms* (q.v.).

mental retardation: Lacking in intelligence, from birth or childhood, to a degree that interferes with a reasonable adjustment in social performance. Emotional conflict often complicates the condition. The need for institutional treatment and care is proportional to the degree of impairment and the level of emotional adjustment. There are four degrees of severity: *mild* (IQ 50-70); *moderate,* (IQ 35-49); *severe,* (IQ 20-34); *profound,* (IQ below 20).

mescaline: An alkaloid originally derived from the peyote cactus, resembling amphetamine and adrenalin chemically used experimentally to produce hallucinations. Used by Indians of the Southwest in religious rites.

mesmerism: Early term for *hypnosis* (q.v.). Named after *Anton Mesmer* (1733-1815).

metapsychology: A psychological theory that cannot be verified or disproved by observation or reasoning.

metrazol shock therapy: See under *shock treatment.*

Meyer, Adolf (1866-1950): Distinguished American psychiatrist, long time professor of psychiatry at Johns Hopkins University, who formulated and introduced the concept of *psychobiology* (q.v.).

migraine: An illness characterized by recurrent, severe, and usually one-sided headaches, often associated with nausea vomiting, and visual disturbances. May be due to unconscious emotional conflicts.

milieu therapy: Literally, treatment by environment in a hospital setting. Physical surroundings, equipment, and staff attitudes are designed in such a way as to enhance the effectiveness of other therapies and foster the patient's rehabilitation.

minor epilepsy (petit mal): See under *epilepsy.*

Mitchell, S. Weir (1830-1914): American neurologist who described *causalgia* and developed a once popular "rest cure" for emotional disorders.

mongolism: A variety of congenital mental retardation characterized by severe intellectual defect, abnormal body development and a fold of skin over the inner angles of the eyes giving a "mongoloid" appearance. Also called Down's Syndrome. The condition results from the presence in the individual's cells of an extra small chromosome (trisomy 21).

monoamine oxidase inhibitor (MAOI): A group of antidepressant drugs which appear to ameliorate the emotional

ate by inhibiting certain brain enzymes and raising the level
serotonin (q.v.).

onomania: See *mania*.

oral treatment: A philosophy and technique of treatment
f mental hospital patients which prevailed in the first half
f the nineteenth century. It emphasized removal of re-
raints, humane and kindly care, attention to religion, and
erformance of useful tasks in the hospital. Historically, the
ntecedent of the modern *therapeutic community* (q.v.).

oron: See *mental retardation*.

otor aphasia: See *aphasia*.

ultiple personality: See *personality, multiple*.

utism: In psychiatry, refusal to speak for conscious or un-
onscious reasons. Often seen in *psychosis*.

ysophobia: See under *phobia*.

n

arcissism (narcism): From Narcissus, figure in Greek my-
hology who fell in love with his own reflected image. Self-
ove, as opposed to object-love (love of another person). In
sychoanalytic theory, cathexis (investment) of the psychic
epresentation of the self with libido (sexual interest and en-
rgy). Some degree of narcissism is considered healthy and

normal; but an excess interferes with relations with others. To be distinguished from egotism, which carries the connotation of self-centeredness, selfishness, and conceit. Egotism is but one expression of narcissism. See also *cathexis, libido*.

narcoanalysis: Similar to narcosynthesis, in which psychotherapy is conducted under the influence of drugs.

narcolepsy: Brief, uncontrollable episodes of sleeping.

narcosis: The sleep-like state induced by a narcotic drug.

narcosynthesis: Psychotherapeutic treatment originally used in acute combat cases under partial anesthesia, e.g., sodium amytal or pentothal.

National Association for Mental Health: Leading voluntary citizen's organization in the mental health field. Founded in 1909 by *Clifford W. Beers* as the National Committee for Mental Hygiene. In 1964 it comprised forty-eight state divisions, one thousand local chapters, and an enrollment of over a million members and volunteers.

necromania: See *mania*.

negative feelings: In psychiatry, hostile, unfriendly feelings.

negativism: Perverse opposition and resistance to suggestions or advice. Often observed in people who subjectively feel "pushed around." Seen normally in late infancy. A common symptom in *catatonic schizophrenia* (q.v. under *schizophrenia*).

neologism: A new word or condensed combination of several words coined by a patient to express a highly complex meaning related to his conflicts; not readily understood by others; common in schizophrenia.

nervous breakdown: A nonmedical, nonspecific term for emotional illness; primarily, a euphemism for psychiatric illness or psychosis.

neurasthenia: A condition marked by symptoms of fatigue, feelings of inadequacy and poor concentration; originally regarded as due to weakness or exhaustion of the nervous system. Obsolescent.

neurologist: A physician with postgraduate training and experience in the field of organic diseases of the nervous system, and whose professional endeavors are primarily concentrated in this area.

neurology: The branch of medical science devoted to the study, diagnosis and treatment of organic diseases of the nervous system.

neuropsychiatry: Combination of the specialties of neurology and psychiatry.

neurosis: See *psychoneurosis*.

night hospital: A hospital, or hospital service, for psychiatric patients who are able to work in the community during the day but who require specialized treatment and supervision in a hospital after working hours.

nightmare (pavor nocturnus): An anxiety dream brought about by massive eruption of repressed sexual and/or aggressive impulses and accompanied by intense anxiety, agonizing dread, a sense of oppression, helpless paralysis, and finally, awakening. In Freud's view, the nightmare represents a failure of the dream work to disguise effectively the unacceptable, unconscious wishes instigating the dream.

nihilism: In psychiatry, the delusion of nonexistence of the self or part of the self.

norepinephrine: The neurohormone of the peripheral sympathetic nervous system. A *catecholamine* related to *epinephrine* (q.v.). Also known as noradrenalin.

nosology: Medical science of classification of diseases.

nymphomania: See *mania*.

O

object relationship: The emotional bonds that exist between an individual and another person as opposed to his interest in, and love for himself; usually described in terms of his capacity for loving and reacting appropriately to others.

obsession: Persistent, unwanted idea or impulse that cannot be eliminated by logic or reasoning.

obsessive compulsive reaction: See under *psychoneurosis*.

obsessive personality: A type of character structure in which there is a pattern of several of the obsessive groups of personality traits or defenses, such as excessive self-imposed orderliness, worry over trifles, indecisiveness, and perfectionism. These may or may not be sufficiently marked to interfere with living, or to limit normal satisfactions and social adjustment.

occupational psychiatry: A special interest field concerned with the diagnosis and prevention of mental illness in industry and with psychiatric aspects of absenteeism, accident proneness, personnel policies, operational fatigue, vocational adjustment, retirement, and related factors.

occupational therapy: An adjunctive therapy commonly used in mental hospitals. It provides opportunity for partial *sublimation* and/or *acting out* (q.v.) of patients' unconscious conflicts and stimulates interests through supervised handicrafts or other activities. Other similar therapies are music, recreation, drama, dance, and bibliotherapy.

oedipus complex (Freud): See under *complex*.

oligophrenia: A term for *mental retardation* (q.v.).

onanism: Incomplete sexual relations with withdrawal just prior to emission. Coitus interruptus. Incorrectly used as a synonym for masturbation.

ntogenic: Pertaining to the biological development of the dividual. Distinguished from *phylogenetic* (q.v.).

pen hospital: Literally, a mental hospital, or section thereof, which has no locked doors or other forms of physical restraint.

perant conditioning: A form of conditioning in which experimental animals or human subjects are trained to operate levers, etc., to obtain rewards or avoid pain. Used extensively in psychiatric and psychopharmacological research.

ral stage: In psychoanalysis, the earliest of the stages of infantile psychosexual development, lasting from birth to 12 months or longer. Usually divided into two phases: the *oral erotic,* related to the pleasurable experience of sucking; and the *oral sadistic,* associated with aggressive biting. Both oral erotism and sadism normally continue in later life in disguised and sublimated forms and may determine certain personality traits.

rganic psychosis: Serious psychiatric disorder resulting from a demonstrable physical disturbance of brain function such as a tumor, infection, or injury. Characterized by impaired memory, orientation, intelligence, judgment, and mood. See also *psychosis.*

rganic disease: Characterized by significant demonstrable structural or biochemical abnormality in an organ or tissue. Sometimes imprecisely used as an antonym for *functional illness* (q.v.).

prientation: Awareness of oneself in relation to time, place, and person.

prienting reflex (OR): Pavlovian term used to describe response to a novel stimulus which is not sufficiently strong to elicit a specific inborn *unconditioned reflex* (q.v.) and which has no background to produce a *conditioned reflex* (q.v.). Turning of the head, focusing of the eyes or ears to a nonspecific noise, light, or touch are examples.

orthopsychiatry: Literally, corrective psychiatry. An approach to the study and treatment of human behavior which involves the collaborative effort of psychiatry, psychology, psychiatric social work, and other behavioral, medical and social sciences in the study and treatment of human behavior

53

in the clinical setting. Emphasis is placed on preventive tech niques to promote healthy emotional growth and develop ment.

overcompensation: A conscious or unconscious process i which a real or fancied physical or psychologic deficit inspire exaggerated correction.

overdetermination: In psychiatry, a term indicating the mu tiple causality of a single emotional reaction or sympton Thus, a single symptom expresses the confluence and conden sation of unconscious drives and needs as well as the defens against them.

overt homosexuality: See under *homosexuality*.

pack: A method of calming and soothing an overactive o agitated psychiatric patient by wrapping him in sheets (usu ally wet but sometimes dry) and then in blankets. Once ex tensively used in most mental hospitals. Now infrequently used.

panic: In psychiatry, an attack of acute, intense, and over whelming anxiety, accompanied by a considerable degree o personality disorganization. See *anxiety*.

panphobia: See under *phobia*.

paranoia: Rare psychotic disorder which develops slowly and becomes chronic. It is characterized by an intricate and nternally logical system of persecutory and/or grandiose delusions. The system stands by itself and does not interfere with the remainder of the personality, which continues apparently intact. To be distinguished from *paranoid schizophrenic reaction* (see under *schizophrenia*) and *paranoid state*.

paranoid: An adjective derived from the noun *paranoia*. Characterized by oversuspiciousness and used to describe any grandiose or persecutory delusions.

paranoid state: Characterized by delusions of persecution which are not so logically systemized as in true *paranoia* (q.v.) nor so bizarre and disorganized as in *schizophrenic reactions*. A paranoid state may be of short duration or chronic.

parapsychology: The study of metapsychic (Psi) phenomena, i.e., the relationship between persons and events which seem to occur extraphysically without the ordinary use of the physical senses. Examples: predicting outcome of throw of dice. See also *psychokenesis* and *extrasensory perception (E.S.P.)*.

paresthesia: Abnormal tactile sensation. Often described as burning, pricking, tickling, tingling, or creeping. May be hallucinatory in certain psychoses or a manifestation of neurological disease.

parasympathetic nervous system: That portion of the *autonomic nervous system* innervating the viscera, glands, blood vessels, etc., which is generally inhibitory and *cholinergic* (q.v.) in function (e.g. vagus nerve).

parataxic distortion: See under *distortion*.

paresis: Weakness of organic origin; incomplete paralysis; term often used instead of *general paresis* (q.v.).

parole (parolee): In psychiatry, technical term for the conditional release of a patient from a mental hospital prior to formal discharge so that the patient may be returned to the hospital if necessary without legal action. Obsolescent because of its association with parole from prison. Similar in meaning to "trial visit," "on leave," and "home leave."

passive-aggressive personality: Characterized by aggressive behavior exhibited in passive ways, such as pouting, stubbornness, procrastination, and obstructionism. May be con sidered a *character disorder* (q.v.).

passive-dependent personality: Characterized by lack o self-confidence, indecisiveness, and emotional dependency May be considered a form of *character disorder*.

pastoral counseling: The use of psychological principles by clergymen in interviews with parishioners who seek help with emotional problems.

pathognomonic: A general medical term which is applied to a symptom or group of symptoms that are specifically diag nostic or typical of a disease entity. Similar to *syndrome* (q.v.)

Pavlov, Ivan Petrovich (1849-1936): Russian neurophysiolo gist noted for his experimental work in the field of *condi tioned reflexes* (q.v.). Awarded Nobel Prize in Medicine (1904) for his work on the physiology of digestion.

pavor nocturnus: See *nightmare*.

pederasty: Homosexual intercourse between man and boy by anus. See also *sodomy*.

penis envy: Literally, envy by the female of the penis of the male. More generally, the female wish for male attri butes, position, or advantages. Believed by many to be a sig nificant factor in female character development.

perception: The mental mechanism by which the nature and/or the meaning of a sensory stimulus or aggregate of stimuli is recognized. It occurs through the use of the senses to integrate and interpret past experiences in response to a present stimulus.

perseveration: Involuntary and pathological persistence of a single response or idea in reply to various questions. Seen most often in organic brain disease.

persona: A Jungian term for the personality mask or facade which each person presents to the outside world. Distin guished from the person's inner being or *anima* (q.v.). See also *Jung*.

personality: The sum total of the individual's internal and external patterns of adjustment to life.

personality disorder: A generic term denoting those mental conditions in which the basic disorder lies in the personality the individual. There is minimal subjective anxiety and tle or no sense of distress. For example, the terms *passive-gressive personality* (q.v.) and *compulsive personality* fall to this category. See also *character disorder; psychopathic rsonality*.

ersonality, multiple: A term used by *Morton Prince* for a re type of dissociative reaction in which the individual lopts two or more different personalities. These are separate and compartmentalized, with total amnesia for the one, ones, not in awareness.

ersuasion: In psychiatry, a therapeutic approach based on rect suggestion and guidance intended to influence favorably patients' attitudes, behavior, and goals.

erversion: Sexual deviation.

etit mal: See *epilepsy*.

hallic stage: The period of psychosexual development from he age of about 2½ to 6 years during which sexual interst, curiosity, and pleasurable experience center about the enis, and in girls, to a lesser extent, the clitoris. See also *ral stage, anal erotism, latency period*.

hantasy: See *fantasy*.

hantom limb: A phenomenon frequently experienced by amutees in which sensations, often painful, appear to originate the amputated extremity.

henothiazine: A chemical originally used as a vermifuge. In sychiatry, a term applied to a group of tranquilizers (e.g. hlorpromazine) which resemble phenothiazine in molecular tructure.

henylketonuria: See *phenylpyruvic oligophrenia*.

henylpyruvic oligophrenia: A congenital metabolic disurbance characterized by an inability to convert phenyllanine to tyrosine. Results in abnormal chemicals which interfere with brain development. Transmitted genetically and reatable by diet when detected in infancy by testing the urine for the presence of phenylpyruvic acid. If untreated, nental retardation results. Also known as phenylketonuria.

hobia: An obsessive, persistent, unrealistic fear of an external object or situation. The fear is believed to arise through a process of displacing an internal (unconscious) conflict to an external object symbolically related to the conflict. (See also *displacement*.) Some of the common phobias are:

acrophobia: Fear of heights.

agoraphobia: Fear of open places.

ailurophobia: Fear of cats.

algophobia: Fear of pain.

claustrophobia: Fear of closed spaces.

mysophobia: Fear of dirt and germs.

panphobia: Fear of everything.

xenophobia: Fear of strangers.

phobic reaction: See under *psychoneurosis*.

phrenology: Abandoned theory of relationship between bone structure of the skull and mental traits.

phylogenetic: Pertaining to the evolutionary or racial history of the species. See also *ontogenic*.

pica: A craving for unnatural food; a perverted appetite. Example: children eating plaster or dirt. Seen in hysteria, pregnancy, and emotionally disturbed children.

Pick's disease. A presenile degenerative disease of the brain affecting the cerebral cortex, particularly the frontal lobes. Symptoms include intellectual deterioration, emotional instability, and loss of social adjustment. See also *Alzheimer disease,* which is similar.

Pinel, Phillipe (1746-1826): French physician-reformer who pioneered in abolishing the use of restraints in the care of the mentally ill.

placebo: Originally, an inactive substance given to "placate" a patient who demands medication (e.g. a "bread pill"). In modern usage, a pharmacologically inert substance administered for therapeutic or experimental reasons because of its potential psychological effect. May be therapeutic or noxious in its effect due to suggestion by the therapist or experimenter or due to the patient's self-induced expectation (faith, fear, apprehension, hostility, etc.). In British usage placebo is sometimes called a "dummy."

play therapy: A treatment technique utilizing the child's play as a medium for expression and communication between patient and therapist.

leasure principle: The basic psychoanalytic concept that nan instinctually seeks to avoid pain and discomfort, and trives for gratification and pleasure. In personality development theories the pleasure principle antedates and subsequently comes in conflict with the *reality principle* (q.v.).

olyphagia: Pathological overeating.

orphyria: An episodic metabolic disorder characterized by he excretion of porphyrins in the urine and accompanied by ttacks of abdominal pain, peripheral neuropathy, and acute sychotic manifestations.

ositive feeling: In psychiatry, warm, friendly feelings, as pposed to negative, hostile feelings.

ostpartum psychosis: A psychotic episide following childbirth; usually schizophrenic in nature. Organic and/or toxic nfluences may be present.

potency: In psychiatry, the male's ability to carry out sexual relations. Often used to refer specifically to the capacity to have and maintain adequate erection of the penis during sexual intercourse.

preconscious: Referring to thoughts which are not in immediate awareness, but which can be recalled by conscious effort.

prefrontal lobotomy: A type of *psychosurgery* (q.v.).

pregenital: In psychoanalysis, refers to the period of early childhood before the genitals have begun to exert the predominant influence in the organization or patterning of sexual behavior. Oral and anal influences predominate during this period. See also *oral stage, anal erotism*.

primal scene: In psychoanalytic theory, the real or fancied observation by the infant of parental or other heterosexual intercourse.

primary gain: A term used in connection with neurotic symptoms. The basic internal psychologic gain of an emotional illness. The concept is that mental symptoms, both normal and psychopathologic, develop defensively in largely unconscious endeavors to cope with or to resolve unconscious conflicts. Such symptoms are characteristically the result of a compromise between a pleasure-seeking, instinctual wish and an opposing, moral prohibition which has created an unconscious conflict. Primary gain refers to the element of unconsciou gratification provided by the compromise (symptom) as wel as to the lessening of guilt and fear which it provides. Al mental mechanisms operate in the service of the primary gain, and the need for such gain may be thought of as re sponsible for the initiation of an emotional illness. In contra distinction, the *secondary gain* (q.v.) is that which is secured from a symptom or illness which is already established. Se *mental mechanism.*

primary process: In psychoanalytic theory, the generally unorganized mental activity characteristic of unconscious mental life. Seen in less disguised form in infancy and in dreams. It is marked by the free discharge of *psychic* energy and excitation without regard to the demands of environ ment, reality, or logic. See also *secondary process.*

Prince, Morton (1854-1929): American psychiatrist and neurologist known for his work on "multiple personalities."

prison psychosis: Term for emotional reactions of psychotic depth precipitated by actual or anticipated incarceration.

process schizophrenia: See under *schizophrenia.*

projection: A defense mechanism, operating unconsciously whereby that which is emotionally unacceptable in the self is unconsciously rejected and attributed (projected) to others The attributes so assigned to another are real to the self and the self reacts accordingly.

projective tests: Psychological tests used as a diagnostic too in which the test material is so unstructured that any respons will reflect a projection of some aspect of the subject's under lying personality and psychopathology. Among the most common projective tests are the *Rorschach* (inkblot) and the *Thematic Apperception Test (TAT)* (q.v.).

psychasthenia: Largely obsolete term introduced by *Janet* (q.v.) to include obsessions, compulsions, doubts, feelings of inadequacy and phobias. See also *neurasthenia.*

psychedelic: An adjective most commonly used with refer ence to pharmacological agents which affect the psyche. See also *psychopharmacology.*

psychiatric illness: See *mental disorder.*

psychiatrist: A doctor of medicine with postgraduate training and experience in mental and emotional disorders.

psychiatry: The medical science which deals with the origin, diagnosis, prevention, and treatment of mental and emotional disorders. It also includes such special fields as mental retardation, the emotional components of physical disorders, mental hospital administration, and the legal aspects of psychiatric disorders. See also *descriptive psychiatry; dynamic psychiatry.*

psychic determinism: See *determinism.*

psychic energizer: A popular term for drugs which stimulate or elevate the mood of a depressed patient.

psychoanalysis: A psychologic theory of human development and behavior, a method of research, and a system of psychotherapy, originally described by Sigmund Freud. Through analysis of free associations and interpretation of dreams, emotions and behavior are traced to the influence of repressed instinctual drives and defenses against them in the unconscious. Psychoanalytic treatment seeks to eliminate or diminish the undesirable effects of unconscious conflicts by making the patient aware of their existence, origin, and inappropriate expression in current emotions and behavior.

psychoanalyst: A psychiatrist with additional training in psychoanalysis, who employs the techniques of psychoanalytic therapy.

psychobiology: The school of psychology and psychiatry originated by *Meyer* based on the concept of the individual as a whole biological unit in which total personality development and functioning from birth is studied biographically. Assets and liabilities of the personality are identified and through the process of *distributive analysis* effort is made to effect better utilization of the individual's assets and diminution of his liabilities.

psychodrama: A technique of group psychotherapy in which individuals dramatize their emotional problems.

psychodynamics: The systematized knowledge and theory of human behavior and its motivation, the study of which depends largely upon the functional significance of emotion. Psychodynamics recognizes the role of unconscious motivation in human behavior. It is a predictive science, based on the assumption that a person's total make-up and probable reactions at any given moment are the product of past interactions between his specific genic endowment and the environment in which he has lived from conception onward.

psychogenesis: Production or causation of a symptom or illness by mental or psychic factors as opposed to organic ones.

psychokinesis: The theory that directed thought processes can influence an event, as, for example, by determining what number will show in a throw of dice. See also *parapsychology* and *extrasensory perception (E.S.P.).*

psychologist: One who specializes in psychology. Generally holds a graduate Ph.D. or M.A. degree. Not to be confused with the *psychiatrist* who holds an M.D. and is eligible for medical licensure.

psychologist, clinical: A psychologist with a graduate degree (usually Ph.D.) and with further training in a medical setting, who specializes in research and/or diagnosis and psychotherapy in the field of mental and emotional disorders. Generally, qualified clinical psychologists work in collaboration with psychiatrists and other physicians.

psychology: An academic discipline, a profession, and a science dealing with the study of mental processes and behavior in man and animal. Not to be confused with the medical specialty of *psychiatry.*

psychology, analytic (Jung): See *analytic psychology.*

psychology, individual (Adler): See *individual psychology.*

psychometry: The science of testing and measuring mental and psychologic ability, efficiency, potentials, and functioning including psychopathologic components. An example is the Stanford-Binet test for intelligence.

psychomotor epilepsy: See under *epilepsy.*

psychomotor excitement: Generalized physical and emotional overactivity in response to internal and/or external stimuli as in a hypomanic state.

psychomotor retardation: A generalized retardation of physical and emotional reactions. The opposite of *psychomotor excitement* (q.v.).

psychoneurosis (psychoneurotic disorders): Emotional maladaptations due to unresolved unconscious conflicts. One of the two major categories of emotional illness, the other being the *psychoses* (q.v.). A neurosis is usually less severe than a psychosis, with minimal loss of contact with reality. Thinking and judgment may be impaired. A neurotic illness represents the attempted resolution of unconscious emotional conflicts in a manner that handicaps the effectiveness of a person in living. Types of neuroses are usually classified according to the particular symptoms which predominate. Common types are:

anxiety reaction: Characterized primarily by direct experiencing of anxiety, which may have an acute or gradual onset, with subjective uneasiness or apprehension out of proportion to any apparent external cause. The anxiety is uncontrollable, and the utilization of various specific defense mechanisms common in other neuroses is minor.

conversion reaction (somatic conversion): A reaction in which unacceptable unconscious impulses are converted into bodily symptoms. Instead of being experienced consciously, the emotional conflict is expressed by physical symptoms. In a broad sense, all neurotic reactions may be regarded as somatic, physiologic, or psychologic "conversion," but technically the term is usually restricted to its somatic aspects.

depressive reaction: A general term covering various types of neurotic depressive reactions in which insight is impaired but not so severely as in a psychotic depression. A neurotic depression may progress to a psychotic depression. See *depression*.

dissociative reaction: A reaction characterized by such dissociated behavior as amnesia, fugues, sleepwalking, and dream states. Superficially, sometimes resembles schizophrenia. See also *dissociation*.

obsessive compulsive reaction: Reaction patterns associated with the intrusion of insistent, repetitive, and unwanted ideas, or of repetitive, unwelcome impulses to perform certain acts. The afflicted person may feel compelled to carry out rituals such as repeated hand-washing, touching, or counting.

phobic reaction: A reaction characterized by a continuing, specific, irrational fear out of proportion to apparent stimuli. See *phobia*.

psychoneurotic disorders: See *psychoneurosis.*

psychopathic personality (psychopath): A person whose behavior is predominantly amoral or antisocial and characterized by impulsive, irresponsible actions satisfying only immediate and narcissistic interests without concern for obvious and implicit social consequences accompanied by minimal outward evidence of anxiety or guilt. The term "psychopath" is considered unsatisfactory by many but is still used. See also *sociopath.*

psychopathology: The study of the significant causes and processes in the development of mental illness. In general, synonymous with *psychogenesis* (q.v.).

psychopharmacology: The study of the action of drugs on the psyche.

psychophysiologic disorders: (Psychophysiologic, autonomic and visceral disorders). A term first used in the *1952 Diagnostic and Statistical Manual of Mental Disorders* to replace the term "psychosomatic disorders." Refers to serious disturbances of any organ system caused by prolonged, unresolved emotional conflict.

psychosexual development: The changes and stages which characterize the development of the psychological aspect of sexuality during the period from birth to adult life. Synonym: libidinal development. See also *libido.*

psychosis: A major mental disorder of organic and/or emotional origin in which there is a departure from normal patterns of thinking, feeling, and acting. Commonly characterized by loss of contact with reality, distortion of perception, regressive behavior and attitudes, diminished control of elementary impulses and desires, abnormal mental content including delusions and hallucinations. Chronic and generalized personality deterioration may occur. A majority of patients in public mental hospitals are psychotic.

psychosomatic: Adjective to denote the constant and inseparable interaction of the *psyche* (mind) and the *soma* (body). Most commonly used to refer to illnesses in which the manifestations are primarily physical with at least a partial emotional etiology. See also *psychophysiologic disorders.*

sychosurgery: Treatment of chronic, severe, and intractable psychiatric disorders by surgical removal or interruption of certain areas or pathways in the brain, especially in the prefrontal lobes.

psychotherapy: The generic term for any type of treatment which is based primarily upon verbal or nonverbal communication with the patient in distinction to the use of drugs, surgery, or physical measures such as electro- or insulin shock, hydrotherapy, and others. Most physicians regard intensive psychotherapy as a medical responsibility.

psychotomimetic: Literally, mimicking a psychosis. Used to refer to certain drugs such as LSD (lysergic acid diethylamide) or mescaline which produce psychotic-like states.

psychotropic: Having an affinity for or special action on the psyche, as "psychotropic drug."

puerperal psychosis: See *postpartum psychosis.*

pyromania: See *mania.*

pyromaniac: One who suffers from pyromania; a "firebug."

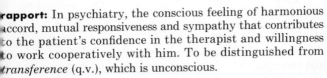

r

rapport: In psychiatry, the conscious feeling of harmonious accord, mutual responsiveness and sympathy that contributes to the patient's confidence in the therapist and willingness to work cooperatively with him. To be distinguished from *transference* (q.v.), which is unconscious.

65

rationalization: A defense mechanism, operating unconsciously, in which the individual attempts to justify or make consciously tolerable, by plausible means, feelings, behavior and motives which would otherwise be intolerable. Not to be confused with conscious evasion or dissimulation. See also *projection.*

Ray, Isaac (1807-81): A founder of the American Psychiatric Association whose "Treatise on the Medical Jurisprudence of Insanity" was the pioneer American work in this field.

reaction formation: A defense mechanism, operating unconsciously, wherein attitudes and behavior are adopted which are the opposites of impulses the individual harbors either consciously or unconsciously—e.g., excessive moral zeal may be a reaction to strong but repressed asocial impulses.

reactive depression: A neurotic depressive reaction apparently precipitated by actual loss of a love object.

reality-principle: In psychoanalytic theory, the concept that the *pleasure-principle* (q.v.), which represents the claims of instinctual wishes, is normally modified by the inescapable demands and requirements of the external world. In fact, the reality-principle may still work in behalf of the pleasure-principle; but it reflects compromises in the nature of the gratification and allows for the postponement of gratification to a more appropriate time. The reality-principle usually becomes more prominent in the course of development, but may be weak in certain psychiatric illnesses and undergo strengthening during treatment.

recall: The process of bringing a memory into consciousness. In psychiatry, recall is often used to refer to the recollection of facts or events in the immediate past.

reference, delusion of, or **idea of:** See *ideas of reference.*

regression: The partial or symbolic return under conditions of relaxation or stress to more infantile patterns of reacting. Manifested in a wide variety of circumstances such as normal sleep, play, severe physical illness, and in many psychiatric disorders.

remission: Abatement of an illness.

repetition compulsion: In psychoanalytic theory the impulse to reenact earlier emotional experiences. Considered by

Freud more fundamental than the *pleasure-principle* (q.v.). According to Ernest Jones: "The blind impulse to repeat earlier experiences and situations quite irrespective of any advantage that doing so might bring from a pleasure-pain point of view."

repression: A defense mechanism, operating unconsciously, which banishes unacceptable ideas, affects, or impulses, from consciousness or which keeps out of consciousness what has never been conscious. Although not subject to voluntary recall, the repressed material may emerge in disguised form. Sometimes used as a generic term for all *defense mechanisms*. Often confused with the conscious mechanism of *suppression*.

resident: An M.D. who has completed his internship and who is in graduate training to qualify as a specialist in a particular field of medicine, such as psychiatry. The American Board of Psychiatry and Neurology requires three years of psychiatric residency training in an approved hospital or clinic together with two years of practice in the specialty of psychiatry to qualify for examination.

resistance: In psychiatry, the individual's conscious and/or unconscious psychological defense against bringing repressed (unconscious) thoughts to light. See also *mental mechanism*.

retardation: Slowing down of mental and physical activity. Most frequently seen in severe depressions which are sometimes spoken of as retarded depressions. Also a synonym for *mental retardation* (q.v.).

retrograde amnesia: See *amnesia*.

retrospective falsification: Unconscious distortion of past experiences to conform to present emotional needs.

rigidity: In psychiatry, refers to an individual's excessive resistance to change.

ritual: In psychiatry, any psychomotor activity sustained by an individual to relieve anxiety. Most commonly seen in *obsessive compulsive neurosis* (q.v.).

RNA: Abbreviation for *ribonucleic acid*. A vital nucleic acid manufactured by *DNA* (q.v.). Essential for the building of body proteins from amino acids. Appears to play a key role in memory.

Rorschach test: A psychologic test developed by the Swiss psychiatrist, Hermann Rorschach (1884-1922), which seeks to disclose conscious and unconscious personality traits and emotional conflicts through eliciting the patient's associations to a standard set of ink-blots.

Rush, Benjamin (1745-1813): Early American physician, signer of the Declaration of Independence, and author of the first American text on psychiatry (1812). He is called "the father of American psychiatry."

S

sadism: Pleasure derived from inflicting physical or psychologic pain on others. The sexual significance of sadistic wishes or behavior may be conscious or unconscious. The reverse of *masochism* (q.v.).

satyriasis: Pathologic or exaggerated sexual drive or excitement in the male. May be of psychic or organic etiology. Analogous to *nymphomania* (q.v.) in the female.

schizoid: Adjective describing traits of shyness, introspection, and introversion.

schizophrenia: A severe emotional disorder of psychotic depth characteristically marked by a retreat from reality with delusion formation, hallucinations, emotional disharmony, and regressive behavior. Formerly called *dementia praecox*. Some types of schizophrenia are:

   ambulatory schizophrenia: Term used by Zilboorg for a schizophrenic who succeeds for the most part in avoiding institutionalization.

catatonic type: Characterized by marked disturbances in activity, with either generalized inhibition or excessive activity. See *catatonia*.

childhood schizophrenia: The somewhat rare onset of schizophrenic reactions in childhood.

hebephrenic type: Characterized by shallow, inappropriate emotions and unpredictable childish behavior and mannerisms.

latent type: A pre-existing susceptibility for developing overt schizophrenia under strong emotional stress or deprivation.

paranoid type: Characterized predominantly by delusions of persecution and/or *megalomania*. See *delusion*.

process schizophrenia: Term used to indicate those forms of severe schizophrenic disorders in which organic brain changes are considered to be the primary cause.

pseudoneurotic type: A form of schizophrenia in which the underlying psychotic process is masked by complaints ordinarily regarded as neurotic.

schizo-affective type: Cases in this category show significant mixtures of schizophrenic and affective (manic-depressive) symptoms.

simple type: Characterized by withdrawal, apathy, indifference and impoverishment of human relationships, but rarely by conspicuous *delusions* or *hallucinations*. It is slowly and insidiously progressive and tends to be unresponsive to current treatments.

scotoma: In psychiatry, a figurative blind spot in an individual's psychologic awareness.

screen memory: A consciously tolerable memory which unwittingly serves as a cover or "screen" for another associated memory which would be disturbing and emotionally painful if recalled.

second signalling system: Pavlovian term for speech in which words are considered to be the "second signals" capable of producing *conditioned responses* (q.v.).

secondary gain: The external gain which is derived from any illness (e.g., personal attention and service, or monetary gains such as disability benefits). See *primary gain*.

secondary process: In psychoanalytic theory, mental activity and thinking characteristic of the ego and influenced by the demands of the environment. Characterized by organization, systematization, intellectualization and similar processes, leading to logical thought and action in adult life. See also *primary process.*

senile dementia: See *dementia, senile.*

senile psychosis: A mental illness of old age characterized by personality deterioration, progressive loss of memory, eccentricity, and irritability. Sometimes called senile dementia. See *dementia, senile.*

sensorium: Roughly synonymous with consciousness. Includes the special sensory perceptive powers and their central correlation and integration in the brain. A clear sensorium conveys the presence of a reasonably accurate memory together with a correct orientation for time, place, and person.

sensory aphasia: See *aphasia.*

sensory deprivation: See *deprivation, sensory.*

separation anxiety: The fear and apprehension noted in infants when removed from their mothers (or surrogates) or in being approached by strangers. Most marked from 6th to 10th month. In later life, similar reaction may result from removal of significant persons or familiar surroundings.

serotonin: A *biogenic amine* (q.v.) derived from tryptophane. Present in the intestine and the brain. A smooth muscle constrictor or stimulator. May influence nervous system activity.

sexual deviation: Sexual behavior at variance with more or less culturally accepted sexual activities. Includes *homosexuality* (q.v.), *transvestitism* (q.v.), sexual *sadism* (q.v.), and sexually violent (criminal) acts.

shell-shock: Obsolete term, used in World War I to designate a wide variety of psychotic and neurotic disorders presumably due to combat experience. See *conversion reaction, hysteria.*

shock treatment: A form of psychiatric treatment in which electric current, insulin, carbon dioxide, or metrazol is administered to the patient and results in a convulsive or comatose reaction to alter favorably the course of illness. Some common types of shock treatment are:

carbon dioxide therapy: A form of shock treatment in which carbon dioxide is administered by inhalation until profound physiological changes and emotional abreactions result.

electroshock treatment (EST) or **electroconvulsive treatment (ECT):** Use of electric current to produce unconciousness and/or convulsive seizures. Most effective in treatment of depressive reactions. Introduced by Cerletti and Bini in 1938. Modifications are *electronarcosis,* producing narcotic-like states, and *electrostimulation,* which avoids convulsions.

insulin coma treatment: A form of treatment in which insulin is injected in large enough doses to produce profound hypoglycemia (low blood sugar) resulting in deep coma. First used by Manfred Sakel in 1933. Infrequently used in the United States since the advent of *tranquilizers.*

metrazol shock therapy: A form of shock treatment, now rarely used, in which a convulsive seizure is produced by intravenous injection of metrazol (known as cardiazol in Europe). Introduced by L. von Meduna in 1935.

subcoma insulin treatment: A form of treatment by the administration of insulin in which drowsiness or somnolence short of coma is produced.

sibling: Term for a full brother or sister.

sibling rivalry: The competition between *siblings* for the love of a parent or for other recognition or gain.

situational depression: See *depressive reaction* under *psychoneurosis.*

social psychiatry: A special interest field concerned with the application of psychiatry to social problems and issues.

social work: The use of community resources and of the conscious adaptive capacities of individuals and groups to better the adjustment of an individual to his environment, or of the environment to the individual.

social worker, psychiatric: A social worker with a graduate degree in social work who utilizes social work techniques in a psychiatric setting.

sociopath: A recent term now in general use and essentially the same as *psychopathic personality* but also connoting a pathological attitude toward society.

sodomy: Anal intercourse between males. Legally, the term may include other types of perversion such as *bestiality*.

somatic conversion: See *conversion reaction* under *psychoneurosis*.

somatization reactions: See *psychophysiologic disorders*.

somnambulism: Sleepwalking. A dissociated or a fugue-like state, in which the person can move about but otherwise seems asleep. Applied also to some states of hypnosis.

status epilepticus: More or less continuous epileptic seizures. See *epilepsy*.

strephosymbolia: Reversal of symbols found in certain reading and writing disorders mainly in children, without evidence of mental defect. For example: writing d-o-g for g-o-d or vice versa. Often results from a confusion in cerebral hemispheric dominance as, for example, when left-handed children are forced to use their right for eating, writing, etc.

stereotypy: Persistent mechanical repetition of speech or motor activity. Common in schizophrenia.

stress reaction: See *gross stress reaction*.

stupor: In psychiatry, a state in which the individual does not react to his surroundings, and appears to be unaware of them. In catatonic stupor, the unawareness is more apparent than real. See *catatonic state*.

stuttering and stammering: Spasmodic speaking with involuntary halts and repetitions, usually considered of psychogenic origin.

subcoma insulin treatment: See under *shock treatment*.

subconscious: Obsolescent in psychiatry. Formerly used to include the preconscious (what can be recalled with effort) and the *unconscious*.

sublimation: A defense mechanism, operating unconsciously by which instinctual drives, consciously unacceptable, are diverted into personally and socially acceptable channels.

subshock insulin treatment: See *subcoma insulin treatment*. under *shock treatment*.

substitution: A defense mechanism, operating unconsciously, by which an unattainable or unacceptable goal, emotion, or object is replaced by one which is more attainable or acceptable. Comparable to *displacement* (q.v.).

succinylcholine: A potent chemical used intravenously in anesthesia as a skeletal muscle relaxant. Also used prior to electroshock therapy to minimize possibility of fractures.

suggestion: In psychiatry, the process of influencing an individual to accept uncritically an idea, belief, or attitude induced by the therapist.

Sullivan, Harry Stack (1892-1949): American psychiatrist best known for his interpersonal theory of psychiatry in which human behavior and personality development are described in terms of the sum total of the interpersonal relations of the individual.

superego: In psychoanalytic theory, that part of the personality associated with ethics, standards and self-criticism. It is formed by the infant's identification with important and esteemed persons in his early life, particularly parents. The supposed or actual wishes of these significant persons are taken over as part of the child's own personal standards to help form the "conscience." In later life they may become anachronistic and self-punitive, especially in psychoneurotic persons. See also, *ego, id.*

supportive psychotherapy: A technique of psychotherapy which aims to reinforce a patient's defenses and to help him suppress disturbing psychological material. Supportive psychotherapy utilizes such measures as inspiration, reassurance, suggestion, persuasion, counselling and reeducation. It avoids probing the patient's emotional conflicts in depth. It is the treatment of choice for patients too fragile to achieve insight or whose symptoms are not sufficient to warrant intensive psychotherapy.

suppression: The conscious effort to control and conceal unacceptable impulses, thoughts, feelings, or acts.

surrogate: One who takes the place of another; a substitute person. In psychiatry, usually refers to an authority figure who replaces a parent in the emotional feelings of the patient (e.g., father-surrogate, mother-surrogate).

symbiosis: In psychiatry, denotes an advantageous relation ship of two disturbed persons who become dependent on each other.

symbolization: An unconscious mental process operating by association and based on similarity and abstract representa tion, whereby one object or idea comes to stand for another through some part, quality or aspect which the two have in common. The symbol carries in more or less disguised form the emotional feelings vested in the initial object or idea.

sympathetic nervous system: That portion of the autonomic nervous system innervating the viscera, glands, blood vessels etc., which is generally excitatory and *adrenergic* (q.v.) in function (e.g., visceral plexuses).

sympathy: Expression of compassion for another's grief or loss. To be differentiated from *empathy* (q.v.).

symptom: A specific manifestation of a patient's condition indicative of an abnormal physical or mental state. Psychi atric symptoms are often the result of unconscious conflict and may represent in symbolic form an instinctual wish, the defense against such a wish, or a compromise between the two.

syndrome: A configuration of symptoms which occur together and which constitute a recognizable illness. Example: *Ganser's syndrome* (q.v.).

Talion law or principle: A primitive, unrealistic belief, usually unconscious, conforming to the Biblical injunction of an "eye for an eye" and a "tooth for a tooth." In psychoanalysis, the concept and fear that all injury, actual or intended, will be punished in kind—i.e., retaliated.

telepathy: The communication of thought from one person to another without the intervention of physical means. Not yet generally accepted as scientifically valid. See also *extrasensory perception*.

Thematic Apperception Test (TAT): A projective psychological test consisting of a series of drawings suggesting life situations which may be variously interpreted depending on the mood and personality of the subject. See also *projective tests*.

therapeutic community: A term of British origin, now widely used, for a specially structured mental hospital milieu which encourages the patient to function within the range of social norms. Special educational techniques are used to overcome the patient's dependency needs and to encourage him to assume personal responsibility to speed the social rehabilitation of himself and the group.

tic: An intermittent, involuntary, spasmodic movement such as a muscular twitch, often without demonstrable external stimulus. A tic may be a disguised expression of a hidden emotional conflict or the result of neurologic disease.

toilet training: The methods used by a child's parents, usually the mother, in teaching and encouraging control of bladder and bowel functions. Occurs at an important period in the formation of the child's personality. Marks the parents' first major effort to control the child and the child's first good chance to resist the parents. Adult attitudes about cleanliness, control, authority and anger arise in part from this period of toilet training and the method by which it is carried out.

topectomy: A type of *psychosurgery* (q.v.).

total push therapy: In a hospital setting, the energetic simultaneous application of all available psychiatric therapies to the treatment of a patient, first described by Abraham Myerson (1881-1948). Myerson emphasized physical activity, recreation, praise, blame, reward, punishment and involvement in care of clothing and personal hygiene.

toxic psychosis: A psychosis resulting from the toxic effect of chemicals and drugs, including those produced in the body. See also *psychosis*.

trance: A state of diminished activity and consciousness resembling sleep. Seen in hypnosis, hysteria, and ecstatic religious states.

tranquilizer: Popular term for any *ataractic* drug (q.v.).

transference: The unconscious "transfer" to others of feelings and attitudes which were originally associated with important figures (parents, siblings, etc.) in one's early life. The transference relationship follows roughly the pattern of its prototype. The psychiatrist utilizes this phenomenon as a therapeutic tool to help the patient understand his emotional problems and their origin. In the patient-physician relationship the transference may be negative (hostile) or positive (affectionate). See also *countertransference*.

transorbital lobotomy: A type of *psychosurgery* (q.v.).

transvestitism (transvestism): Sexual pleasure derived from dressing or masquerading in the clothing of the opposite sex. The sexual origins of transvestitism may be unconscious. There is a strong wish to appear as and to be accepted as a member of the opposite sex.

traumatic neurosis: The term encompasses combat, occupational, and compensation neuroses. These are neurotic reactions which have been attributed to or which follow a situational traumatic event, or series of events. Usually the event has some specific and symbolic emotional significance for the patient, which may be reinforced by *secondary gain* (q.v.).

Tuke, William (1732-1822): English Quaker layman who pioneered in the treatment of patients without physical restraints.

U

ultra-sonotomy: A neurosurgical procedure in the treatment of certain severe psychiatric disorders in which discrete brain lesions are produced (usually in the prefrontal lobes) by the use of ultra sound (high frequency sound waves).

unconditioned reflex (UCR): An inborn physiologic reflex response to an unconditioned stimulus; e.g., salivation at the sight of food.

unconscious: In Freudian theory, that part of the mind or mental functioning the content of which is only rarely subject to awareness. It is repository for data which have never been conscious (primary repression), or which may have become conscious briefly and was then repressed (secondary repression).

underachiever: Term used in child psychiatry for a student who manifestly does not function up to his capacity.

undoing: A primitive defense mechanism, operating unconsciously, in which something unacceptable and already done is symbolically acted out in reverse, usually repetitiously, in the hope of "undoing" it and thus relieving anxiety.

V

vaginismus: Painful vaginal spasm, usually occurring in connection with sexual intercourse.

vegetative nervous system: Obsolescent term for *sympathetic nervous system.*

verbigeration: Stereotyped and seemingly meaningless repetition of words or sentences.

vertigo: Sensation of dizziness, often associated with faintness.

voyeurism: Sexually motivated and often compulsive interest in watching or looking at others, particularly at genitals. Roughly synonymous with "peeping Tom." Observed predominantly in males.

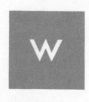

W.A.I.S. (Wechsler Adult Intelligence Scale): A verbal and performance test especially designed to measure intelligence in adults.

waxy flexibility: See *cerea flexibilitas.*

Weyer, Johann (circa 1530): German physician who was one of the first to devote his major interest to psychiatric disorders. Regarded by some as the founder of modern psychiatry.

White, William Alanson (1870-1937): American psychiatrist famous for his early support of psychoanalysis and his contributions to forensic psychiatry.

withdrawal: In psychiatry, a pathological retreat from people or the world of reality, often seen in schizophrenics.

withdrawal symptoms: Term used to describe physical and mental effects of withdrawing drugs from patients who have become habituated or addicted to them.

word salad: A mixture of words and phrases which lack comprehensive meaning or logical coherence, commonly seen in schizophrenic states.

working through: Active exploration of a problem by patient and therapist until a satisfactory solution has been found or until a symptom has been traced to its unconscious sources.

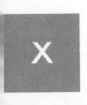

xenophobia: See under *phobia*.